The Mediterranean

FAMILY TABLE

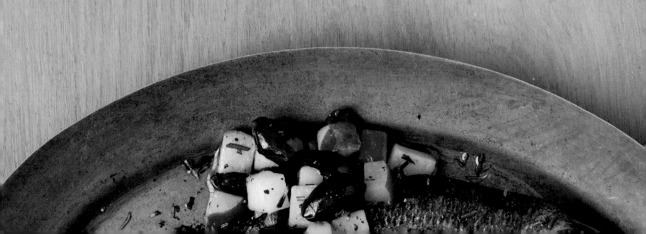

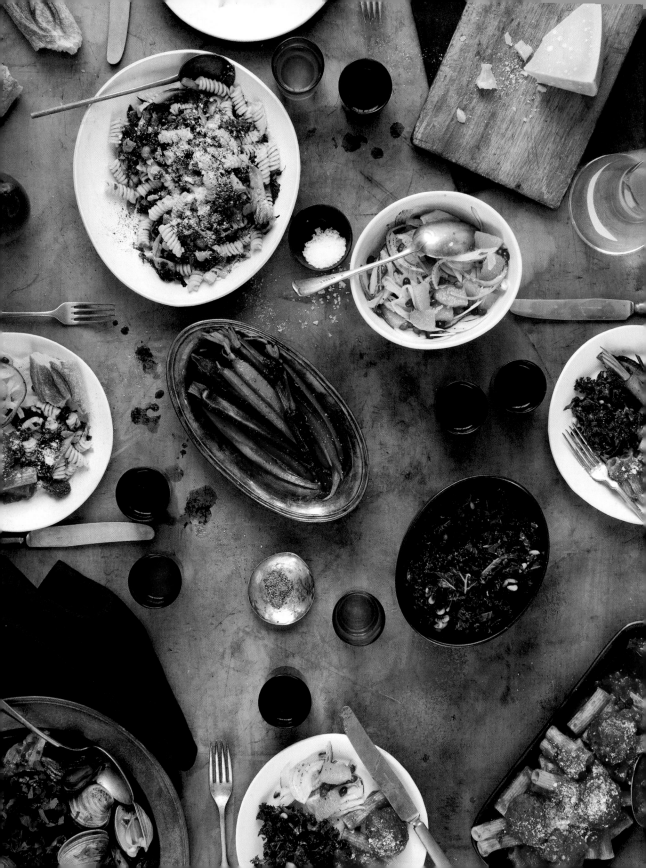

The Mediterranean
FAMILY TABLE

*125 Simple, Everyday Recipes
Made with the Most Delicious and Healthiest Food on Earth*

ANGELO ACQUISTA, M.D.

with Laurie Anne Vandermolen

PHOTOGRAPHY BY LIZ CLAYMAN | STYLING BY REBEKAH PEPPLER

WILLIAM MORROW

An Imprint of HarperCollinsPublishers

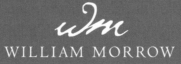

This book is written as a source of information only. The information contained in this book should by no means be considered a substitute for the advice of one's qualified medical professional, who should always be consulted before beginning any new diet, exercise, or other health program.

All efforts have been made to ensure the accuracy of the information contained in this book as of the date published. The author and the publisher expressly disclaim responsibility for any adverse effects arising from the use or application of the information contained herein.

FIRST EDITION

Designed by Suet Yee Chong

Photography by Liz Clayman Photography
Images on pages 235, 244, and 250 courtesy of Svetlana Acquista

Styling by Rebekah Peppler

Library of Congress Cataloging-in-Publication Data has been applied for.

ISBN 978-0-06-240718-4

15 16 17 18 19 OV/RRD 10 9 8 7 6 5 4 3 2 1

To those I have most loved having around my table,
my wife, Svetlana, my children, Alessandra, Salvatore, and Nicholas,
my mother, Sara, and my brother Domenick,
who has always been beside me, as both a brother and a father figure

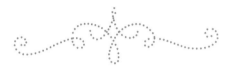

In loving memory of my father,
Salvatore Acquista

Contents

Eat Well

Mangiare Bene

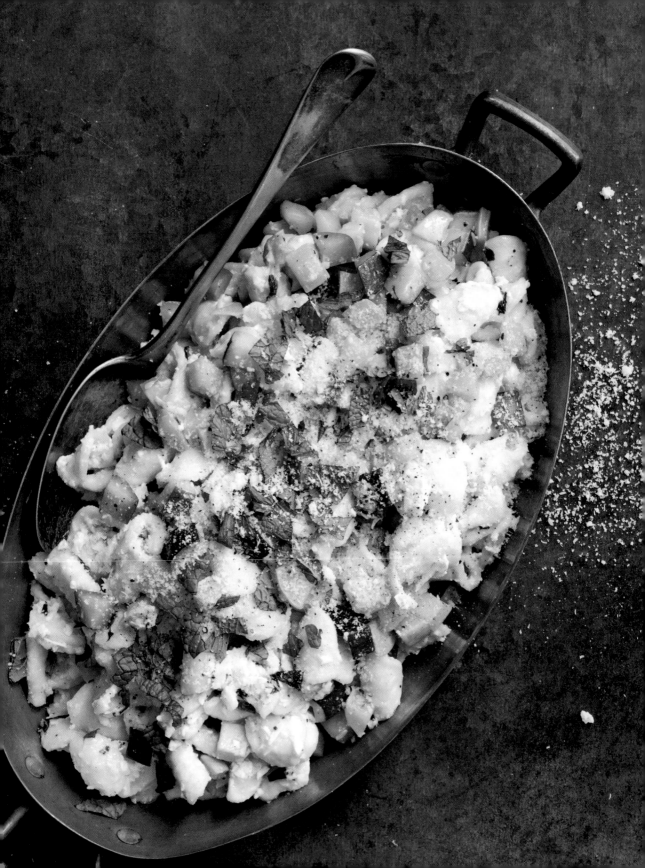

INTRODUCTION

*Tutti a tavola is an Italian phrase I heard almost every day while growing up in Sicily. It means "all to the table." To me this simple, poetic phrase encompasses what this cookbook is all about, and indeed what the Mediterranean diet and lifestyle are all about. Reduced to its elements, the Mediterra-*nean diet is, as its originator, Dr. Ancel Keys, describes, "pasta in many forms, leaves sprinkled with olive oil, all kinds of vegetables in season, and often cheese, all finished off with fruit, and frequently washed down with wine." Olives, nuts, whole grains, and fish are plentiful, legumes like beans are abundant, and meat is scarce. Beyond the dietary heritage of the region, however, the traditions of spending time and sharing meals with friends and family, and cultivating a reverent appreciation for food and its preparation begin in infancy and last a lifetime. These customs embody the Mediterranean way just as much as the menu (and may also play a big part in the many health benefits the diet bestows).

Although many countries with a range of cuisines border the Mediterranean Sea, for our purposes when we use the term "Mediterranean diet," we are talking about the one defined by scientists in terms of health. This means its components reflect food patterns typical of the island of Crete, much of the rest of Greece, and southern Italy in the early 1960s. The selection of this particular time and these geographical areas is mainly based upon two lines of evidence:

1. In Keys's Seven Countries Study conducted at that time, among other research, it was found that life expectancy for populations in these areas was among the highest in the world, and rates of heart disease, other diet-related chronic diseases, and certain cancers were among the lowest in the world, despite limited medical services.
2. In numerous epidemiological studies conducted throughout the world, similar dietary patterns in other populations have also been associated with long life expectancy and low rates of chronic disease.

Hence, "Mediterranean diet" specifically refers to dietary patterns found in these olive-growing areas of the Mediterranean region around fifty years ago.

To my good fortune, I spent my youth in southern Italy during this era. Little did I know at the time that I was eating one of the healthiest diets scientists have ever been able to identify. Sicily is just off the southern coast of Italy, and I lived in Castrofilippo, a small, rural town near the sea. When Keys and others depict the quintessential Mediterranean diet and lifestyle, they are describing the way I grew up.

In general, people were poor, so we grew our own fruits and vegetables, fished the sea, made olive oil from the olive trees in our backyard, made wine from the grapes we grew, picked our own walnuts, made our own bread, and collected eggs from our own chickens. Meat was in short supply. Our lives were centered on our families, and our families were often centered in the kitchen. The kitchen was the heart and soul of the home. It's where everyone of all ages gathered, babies to grandparents.

At mealtimes, everyone ate a version of the same thing. From the time I had teeth and could manage soft food, my mother was taking whatever was on the table and mashing it up with a fork for me. We kids ate local, unprocessed foods that were soft, like fresh figs and peaches, ricotta cheese, and fresh mozzarella. There was daily fresh-baked whole-grain bread that we soaked in dense, aromatic olive oil. We would eat any vegetable on the table. Eventually we would eat the full adult menu, and the older folks who had dental troubles would return to the soft foods of their youth.

The Mediterranean diet is meant to be enjoyed together by the whole family—

say good-bye to short-order cooking—which is why I wrote this book to include all life stages. Starting children at a very early age primes them to have the taste and habits of healthy eating for their entire lives. In fact, in raising my own kids the same way I was raised, even at three and six years old, they will eat anything, even healthy food supposedly only enjoyed by adults. As my six-year-old daughter, Alessandra, says when given a choice at mealtime, "I want to eat what Papa eats." They eat kale, broccoli rabe, Brussels sprouts, figs, salmon, octopus, mackerel, and so on, and they truly enjoy it.

I have included sections for each stage of childhood to address children's diverse nutritional concerns. I have also included a general section for adults (with some attention given to the particular needs of young adults, pregnant women, and those going through middle age and menopause), and a section for the sixty-plus audience looking to maximize health in the golden years (it's never too late to benefit from eating healthfully!).

I have had a long-standing interest in nutrition and weight management in my clinical practice in internal medicine. I have also been cooking for most of my adult life—first during medical school, while my mother advised me over the phone, and eventually taking over and cooking for anyone and everyone in my life. My wife is much more beautiful than I am handsome, but I sealed the deal after I cooked for her. In time, I merged these two interests in my medical practice. When patients were trying to lose weight, I realized that they didn't start following the healthy Mediterranean diet I described until I started writing recipes down on my prescription pad and telling them, "This is the prescription medicine I would like you to try." The approach was so effective for weight loss that it became the topic of my first book, *The Mediterranean Prescription*. While the book was illuminating in telling how to follow the Mediterranean diet and what the science was, readers couldn't seem to get enough of the recipes.

Here in *The Mediterranean Family Table,* I bring you a bounty of Mediterranean recipes to try, savor, and gather around. The southern Italian style is simple—using flavorful ingredients that are varied and fresh—and not particularly fancy. This makes it perfect for you, the modern, busy cook who wants to eat more whole foods, prepare delicious and nourishing meals, and still have time to linger over them with your loved ones.

Buon appetito!

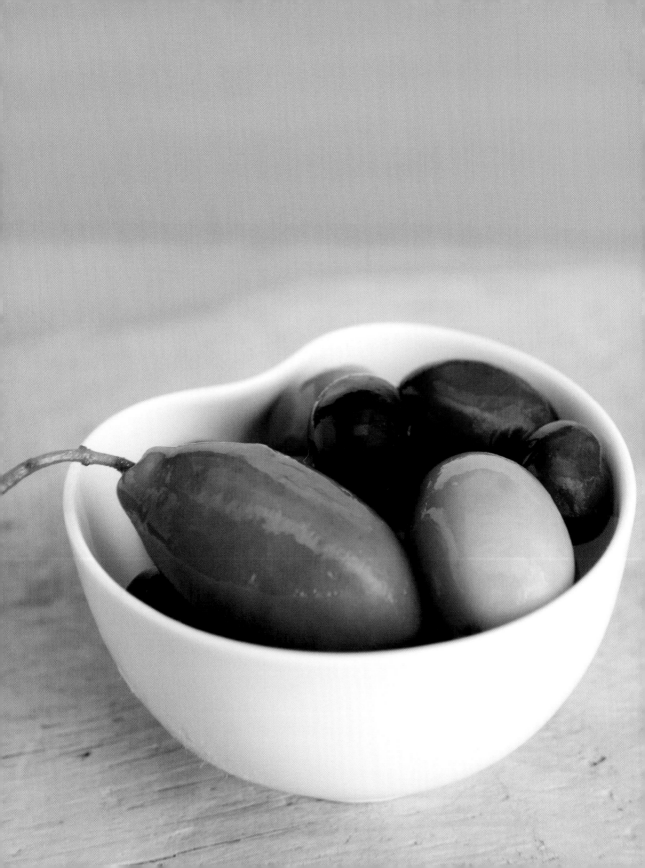

EAT HEALTHY

Mangiare Sano

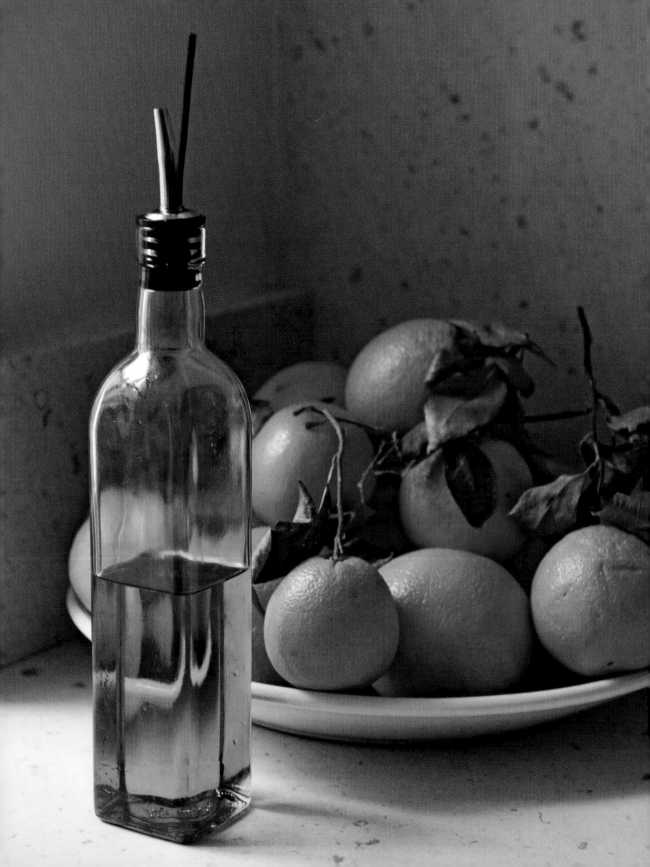

WHAT IS THE
MEDITERRANEAN DIET?

In February 2013, one of the most esteemed medical journals in the world, the New England Journal of Medicine, *published a study on the topic of the Mediterranean diet. It was one of those uncommon diet trials with all of the right parameters: a large number of people were randomly assigned* to groups with specified menus and followed for several years. At the end of a five-year follow-up period, investigators came to a remarkable conclusion—that people who ate a Mediterranean diet drenched in olive oil and laden with nuts had reduced the chance they would suffer a heart attack, stroke, or death attributable to cardiovascular disease *by 30 percent.*

While the Mediterranean diet is best known for its contribution to heart health, by no means do its benefits end there. In fact, in addition to those heart-related illnesses, countless studies have touted the many life-giving benefits of the Mediterranean diet—demonstrating some level of protection from virtually

Why Is Everyone So Concerned About Heart Disease?

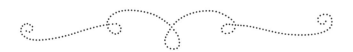

I talk a lot about heart disease prevention in this book. The reason is simply that cardiovascular disease is the number one killer worldwide—it was back in Ancel Keys's time, and it still is today. Here's a rough breakdown of the eight most common ways people died in 2010 in the US:

Heart disease	600,000
Cancer	575,000
Chronic lower respiratory diseases	140,000
Stroke	130,000
Accidents	120,000
Alzheimer's	85,000
Diabetes	70,000
Kidney disease	50,000

At a glance, heart disease and cancer deaths seem comparable. However, when you look at deaths caused by cardiovascular disease—which is responsible for heart disease but also affects the entire circulatory system—they number more than 800,000. This includes heart disease, stroke (90 percent are the clotting type related to the process that causes heart attacks), and many other blood-vessel-related conditions. Diabetes, Alzheimer's, and kidney disease are also thought to be linked to or worsened by cardiovascular disease. Cancer is number two on the list, resulting in around 575,000 deaths. However, of those, 160,000 cases are lung cancer, in which the majority are related to smoking. The next most common cancers are colorectal (50,000 deaths per year), breast (40,000), pancreatic (40,000), and prostate (30,000). Each one of these cancers has its own set of risk factors—such as genetics, diet, environmental toxins, hormones, and various other carcinogens. Cardiovascular disease, in contrast, has a more unified cause, so following its prevention plan has the potential to help most people's greatest risk. Furthermore, the same diet and lifestyle recommendations that help prevent heart and cardiovascular disease generally help protect from cancer—and all of the other major chronic diseases—as well.

all of our most serious and deadly chronic conditions, including cancer, diabetes, Alzheimer's, arthritis, and obesity—since its investigation began around seventy years ago.

Pursuit of an ideal diet began in earnest when heart attacks began increasing at an alarming rate in the 1940s. No health concern was more urgent than heart disease at that time, as it was responsible for around 40 percent of all deaths in the United States (and if you included stroke, which is related to the same disease process, the figure was 50 percent). The overall death rate was much higher then as well, and about half the deaths were caused by a disease of the arteries. Again and again, men in the prime of life were dropping from sudden cardiac death. It wasn't long before the leader of the United States, President Dwight Eisenhower, had a massive heart attack while in office at the age of sixty-five. The nation was on edge and looking for answers.

In 1947, Ancel Keys, the scientist most people think of as the father of the Mediterranean diet, began to look into the problem. Diet had been suggested as a probable cause for heart disease since at least the turn of the twentieth century, but an understanding of the connection remained murky. Cholesterol had been identified as a likely candidate for having something to do with it, singled out because it was found that the arterial clots themselves were glutted with it. When a number of substantial studies came out clearly demonstrating that cholesterol levels in the blood were higher in patients with heart disease, many thought they had at last confirmed the dietary culprit. However, Keys performed studies that showed it was not the cholesterol one *ate* that made it available in the blood to form blockages in the arteries.

Keys had begun to hypothesize what else it might be besides cholesterol in the diet that was causing those high levels, when an unusual patient he happened to examine took him in a novel direction. A sick Wisconsin dairy farmer was referred to him by the University of Wisconsin medical school. As Keys described it, "He had big knobs on his elbows and over his eyes, and when you opened them, it was just pure cholesterol inside." After trying various treatments, Keys's team checked the farmer's blood cholesterol level, and the first reading was sky high—1,000 mg/dL, compared with the average level in the US of 220 or 230. The man's brother had come in with him as well and had a reading of 600. The two were sent to Keys's Minnesota lab, where they stayed and were fed an almost fat-free diet for a week, and "Bang!" as Keys put it, their cholesterol levels dropped down to 500 and 300. Keys contemplated what might happen if he gave them some fat, so he had them eat some vegetable margarine, and sure enough, their cholesterol levels shot back up again. Hence, it appeared that it was *fat* that was affecting their cholesterol levels. It was ultimately the result of this particular investigation that led to his painstaking testing of how fats, in their many forms, could affect health and disease.

Keys went on to perform further feeding studies, which convinced him that, indeed, blood cholesterol levels were the result of how much fat was consumed in the diet. Postwar statistics also revealed an intriguing clue to the mystery. Keys noticed that American business executives, presumably among the best-fed people in the world, had high rates of heart disease, while in postwar Europe, heart disease rates had plummeted in the wake of reduced supplies of foods like meat and dairy. He was also impressed and intrigued by the alleged low rates of heart disease being reported in the Mediterranean region. "Heart disease is no problem here," an Italian colleague had told him. "Come and see for yourself." And so in 1952, he left for Italy.

Keys took a sabbatical as a Senior Fulbright Scholar and settled in Naples. It was a trip that would change him in many ways. From a research standpoint, it was the dawn of collecting international health and nutritional data to compare with other regions. For example, it quickly became clear that cholesterol levels in Naples were much lower than those being measured in America and England; it also soon became clear as he toured Neapolitan hospitals that heart disease in the region was indeed a rarity. Inspired, Keys continued to expand his reach, collecting data from Madrid as well. His reports stimulated an international group to join in, generating measurements and diagnoses in South Africa, Japan, and Finland.

The collective data supported the notion that differing fats in the diet were associated with distinct cholesterol levels in the blood, as well as in the frequency of heart disease. In Japan, for instance, they observed communities with low incidence of heart disease who ate a very low-fat diet, whereas in Finland they encountered farmers and woodcutters, many of them lean and muscular yet suffering from heart disease, who buttered their cheese.

The other transformation Keys experienced in Naples was more subtle and less scientific, at least at the time: he fell in love with the food and culture of southern Italy. An Italian professor, Flamino Fidanza, assisted him not only by procuring facilities and study subjects, but also by hosting him and initiating him into the Neapolitans' way of life. Keys absorbed and embraced their culinary tastes and habits, their tendency to walk everywhere and get out in the sunshine, their tendency to drink a glass or two of wine with supper. This hilly, flower-dappled, seaside introduction would turn out to be just as important as the scientific revelations to come.

In reflecting on the time he spent there, Keys later said, "My concern about diet as a public health program began in the early 1950s in Naples, where we observed very low incidences of coronary heart disease associated with what we later came to call the 'good Mediterranean diet.'" He found that this diet was loaded with fruits, vegetables, and whole grains, differing from American and northern European diets in that it was much lower in meat and dairy products and embraced fruit for dessert. These observations culminated in his development of the Seven Countries Study.

With the active participation of leading international cardiologist Paul Dudley White (President Eisenhower's personal cardiologist), the Seven Countries Study was a meticulously planned and executed ten-year investigation of the epidemiology of coronary disease in sixteen populations of six Western countries and Japan. Around 13,000 men were studied, aged forty to fifty-nine, from Yugoslavia, Finland, Italy, the Netherlands, Greece, the United States, and Japan. It took years of negotiations, fund-raising, planning, and trial runs (the first of these trials were in Crete and southern Italy) before communities began being monitored in 1958. This massive endeavor was a milestone study on numerous counts, marking the first effort in history to leap international borders and compare diet-disease associations between communities with widely differing culinary and lifestyle populations. The hope was that the regional differences in risk, health behavior, and biological factors could be measured, thus providing direction to prevent—or at the very least decelerate—heart disease around the world.

The first results from the Seven Countries Study were published in 1970, after ten years of data collecting. As Keys had predicted, a high amount of fat in the diet—especially saturated fat (the kind found in meat and dairy)—was correlated with heart disease. Both the island of Crete in Greece and southern Italy were heralded as the shining stars of the study, having by far the lowest proportion of heart disease and the longest life expectancy. Americans, by contrast, had a 72 percent greater chance of dying from heart disease than the Italians. It was clear that diet was related, but since only the macronutrient contents were used for analysis (that is, the amounts of proteins, carbohydrates, and fats), the specific foods of the diets were not published for some time.

The Seven Countries Study generated much interest in the eating habits of the healthiest people in the world. Over time, research was published that demonstrated the benefits for the other elements of the Mediterranean diet aside from eating little saturated fat. It turned out that all the antioxidants, vitamins, minerals, fiber, healthy proteins, complex carbohydrates, and wine these people were consuming promoted health and longevity as well.

Throughout the 1980s and 1990s, scientists, nutritionists, and doctors worked to define what the Mediterranean diet was exactly. After all, there are more than fifteen countries that surround the Mediterranean Sea, with overlapping cuisines. Which formula was the best? In the end, they kept coming back to the 1960s rural diets of Crete and southern Italy. In addition, in 1989, one of the directors involved in the Seven Countries Study published a historical record of what the subjects in all of the countries under investigation were eating around the time of the study. The proportions for Crete and southern Italy at that time are now taken to be the ideal healthy Mediterranean diet because of those communities' very low incidence of heart disease and other diet-linked conditions (though their diets and disease rates have since changed). The data were confirmed by other investigations and thus constitute the principal research basis for the proportions of foods in modern Mediterranean diet pyramids.

One of the first clinical trials in support of the restorative health benefits of the Mediterranean diet as a whole, a groundbreaking study known as the Lyon Diet Heart Study, came in 1994. Six hundred patients in France who had had a heart attack were randomly assigned to either a Mediterranean-style diet or a control diet similar to what the American Heart Association recommended for the general population to reduce the risk of heart disease. Two years into the study, the compelling results came in: the Mediterranean group had a 73 percent reduced risk of coronary events and 70 percent reduced overall chance of dying as compared with the control diet. The study was meant to go for five years but was stopped after an interim analysis showed such significant beneficial effects in the patients receiving the Mediterranean diet. Adding to the significance of this study was the intriguing finding that, despite a robust connection between adhering to the Mediterranean diet and living longer, no appreciable associations were seen for the *individual* components of the diet. It was becoming clear that it was the diet *as a whole* that was the best for your overall health and protection from disease.

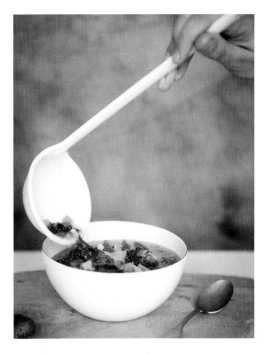

As research continued, it also became apparent that the Mediterranean diet was not just good for your heart. Any condition related to arteries or veins generally benefited. Data from a series of studies have also shown that sticking to the Mediterranean diet is associated with a reduced risk for developing various cancers. The risk of contracting degenerative diseases of the brain such as Parkinson's and Alzheimer's appears to be reduced as well. It has also been related to lower body fat and lower incidence of diabetes. Moreover, the Mediterranean diet has long been recognized to reduce mortality overall.

By the year 2000, the quantity of fat in the diet came under scrutiny, challenging many deeply held beliefs that a low-fat diet was the ideal. It was acknowledged that, even though high amounts of fat in the diet were linked to heart disease, some of the regions the Mediterranean diet were modeled after actually had a high fat content in their diet, up to around 40 percent of their daily calories. But it wasn't saturated fat they had been eating—their diet had olive oil poured all over it. With a combination of monounsaturated fat and antioxidants that benefit health in numerous ways, olive oil seemed to be an essential health elixir, helping to thwart disease in many shapes and forms.

The International Task Force for Prevention of Coronary Disease said in a consensus statement around this time, "There is increasing scientific evidence that there are positive health effects from diets which are high in fruits, vegetables, legumes, and whole grains, and which include fish, nuts, and low-fat dairy products. Such diets need not be restricted in total fat as long as there is not an excess of calories, and should emphasize predominantly vegetable oils that are low in saturated fats and partially hydrogenated oils [trans fats, found in many commercially processed foods]. The traditional Mediterranean diet, whose principal source of fat is olive oil, encompasses all of these dietary characteristics."

An interdisciplinary, multicultural conference was held in Rome to further update and standardize the Mediterranean diet in 2005. The participants invoked an ancient Greek word, *ataraxia*—which connotes "equilibrium," "lifestyle," and being in a state of robust tranquillity while surrounded with trustworthy and affectionate friends—to accompany the description of the Mediterranean diet. In presenting it as more than just a diet, they recognized the importance of the entire lifestyle upon health and well-being. Physical, social, and culinary activities also play an essential role.

So where are we now? Scientists have not yet found a magic bullet for health, probably because one doesn't exist—our bodies are far too complicated for that. However, at this point in history, it appears we have identified the diet of the people who have the least disease and live the longest. Perhaps the magic is that the Mediterranean diet improves universal biological features that promote health, such as reducing inflammation and excess body fat; perhaps it's the timing of consuming antioxidants within the food during the course of the meal; perhaps it's the environment of warm social connection enjoyed by the healthiest communities; perhaps it's that a diet so fresh, varied, and delicious, yet simple, is so easy to take on. It is most certainly partly all of these things.

WHAT MAKES THE MEDITERRANEAN DIET SO GOOD FOR YOU?

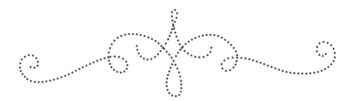

Following World War II, the rural people of Crete and southern Italy probably developed their menus and way of life out of necessity rather than choice. However, in living off the land and sea, concentrating on fresh and unprocessed food, and not eating much meat or dairy, these Mediterranean communities inadvertently ate a diet that consisted of healthy fats, proteins, and whole grains and was loaded with fiber, vitamins, minerals, antioxidants, and phytochemicals—with one meal a day often washed down with a relaxing glass of wine. The focus on fresh food maximized nutrients and minimized processing, which generally strips out the good-for-you parts and adds in unhealthy fats, sugars, and chemicals. Eating a wide variety of food as they did also ensured an array of nutrients while reducing exposure to any one toxin. This combination seems to be largely responsible for the remarkable healthfulness of the Mediterranean diet.

A Closer Look at Cholesterol, the Good and the Bad

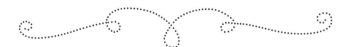

Many people mistakenly believe that cholesterol slowly builds up in the arteries until it blocks blood flow like clogged pipes in a kitchen sink. However, the cholesterol pileup is actually happening *inside* the lining of the arteries. As cholesterol accumulates there, it will narrow and stiffen the walls of the arteries, increasing blood pressure. Unstable plaques will eventually burst and cause a blood clot to form at the rupture site. These clots can cut blood flow on the spot or after traveling to distant arteries and are responsible for the vast majority of heart attacks, as well as strokes.

Cholesterol's journey into the walls of the arteries to form into plaques is made possible by lipoproteins, which cholesterol requires to escort it around. There's actually only one kind of cholesterol—when we say "good" or "bad" cholesterol, we're really talking about good or bad *lipoproteins,* because they determine where the cholesterol goes. It turns out that lipoproteins' density is related to their function.

High-density lipoprotein (HDL) trolls around the circulatory system looking for cholesterol passengers, shuttling them back to the liver for your body to recycle or eliminate, so it's thought of as the "good" kind. Low-density lipoprotein (LDL), on the other hand, delivers cholesterol around the body, such as to cells that require more than they're able to make for themselves; however, too much LDL causes damage, so it's thought of as the "bad" kind. LDL tends to get deposited and taken up into the walls of the arteries, especially damaged vessel walls, which can promote a never-ending cycle of inflammation and more deposits. And the more LDL you have, the more cholesterol is available to be delivered there.

The degree to which LDL gets oxidized within arterial walls also accounts for its danger to health. So much so that LDL oxidation may even be a better marker for cardiovascular risk than any other, though at this time LDL oxidation is very difficult and expensive to measure.

Diet is involved because it affects LDL and HDL levels and because the kinds of fat in the diet affect how much LDL gets oxidized.

In the following pages I'll describe what it is about the nature of the food that makes it so good for your weight and health. Then, I'll briefly explain how this pattern of eating enables optimal functioning throughout your body, which is what provides you with strength and energy, slows down the aging process, and keeps so many common chronic conditions and diseases away.

HEALTHY FOODS, HEALTHY BODY

Unquestionably, the **fat makeup** of the Mediterranean diet is paramount to its promotion and protection of health. The dominance of monounsaturated fat, namely in the form of olive oil, imparts countless health benefits. Polyunsaturated omega-3 fats, as well as polyunsaturated omega-6 fats, are also plentiful and offer many benefits.

The biochemical nature of the monounsaturated, omega-3, and omega-6 fats makes them more fluid in the body (what we want). The unsaturated bonds of these fats have the potential to react with damaging oxygen free radicals (when that happens, it's called oxidation), but because they're usually accompanied by antioxidants—such as the vitamin E found in olives—they are protected from attack. Saturated and trans fats, on the other hand, which are in short supply in the Mediterranean diet, can be stacked tightly, adding unwelcome rigidity to cell membranes and allowing for them to be stored more easily and plentifully in cells.

Olive oil (extra virgin) may have the perfect collective features for a fat: it is a monounsaturated fat, so it has only one unsaturated bond, making it fluid yet not prone to much oxidation, and it contains an unusually large quantity of potent antioxidants and phytonutrients relative to its fat content. Since oxidation of the bad LDL cholesterol looks to be a fundamental step in the development of cardiovascular disease, the fact that olive oil both reduces the quantity of LDL in the blood *and* protects it from oxidation is very important indeed.

The **omega-3 fatty acids** are called "essential fats" because the body doesn't make them, so they need to be ingested. There are three main types: alpha-linolenic acid (ALA), which comes from plant sources like nuts and avocados, and eicosapentaenoic acid (EPA) and docosahexaenoic acid (DHA), which come mostly from fish (hence are sometimes called marine omega-3s). They make blood less likely to form clots inside arteries (the cause of most heart attacks), improve blood cholesterol levels, limit inflammation, and prevent erratic heart rhythms.

Omega-6 fats are also thought to be heart healthy, helping regulate inflammation and blood pressure, as well as heart, gastrointestinal, and kidney functions—in the proper amounts. The ratio of omega-6 fats to omega-3 fats is important. A four-to-one or even one-to-one ratio would be best; however, most people currently consume around 10 to 20 omega-6s to 1 omega-3. Given that the omega-6 soybean oil is used extensively in the commercial food industry, the imbalance of omega-6s to omega-3s can be significantly improved upon if processed food is reduced in the diet.

Whole grains are also a staple of the Mediterranean diet. A whole grain, or seed, naturally comes with three components: the bran or outer shell (with fiber, vitamins, and minerals), the germ (an inner core rich with antioxidants and vitamins B and E), and the endosperm (the majority of which is carbohydrate). Whole grains can be milled into cereals and flour. When grains are refined, however, the healthy bran and germ are removed during processing, and the endosperm is pulverized, leaving behind just an easily digestible calorie-packed carbohydrate. Because the body doesn't digest whole grains as fast, you stay full longer, and blood sugar and insulin levels don't spike. Better control of blood sugar metabolism helps prevent the development of excess weight, diabetes, and heart disease.

Fiber is the indigestible part of plants. It helps regulate bowel function by adding bulk and appears to help sweep harmful substances from the intestines. Fiber also helps to reduce cholesterol levels, control blood sugar by slowing its absorption, promote weight loss by slowing down chewing and digestion, satisfy hunger without extra calories, and keep you feeling full over time. It's also known to reduce the risk of diseases such as heart disease, diabetes, diverticulitis, irritable bowel syndrome, and certain cancers.

Protein has been studied less compared with fats and carbohydrates in terms of its role in the onset of disease, but research suggests that protein from vegetable sources, which the Mediterranean diet emphasizes, is better for you than protein from animal sources. Of note, if you're getting your protein from nuts and legumes, you're also ingesting healthy fats, fiber, and antioxidants. In contrast, if you're getting your protein from beef or dairy products made from whole milk, you are also consuming saturated fat, without those nutritional bonuses.

Another important aspect of the Mediterranean diet is its abundance of **antioxidants**. Antioxidants are the biological heroes that absorb harmful single-oxygen free radicals that would otherwise damage lipids, proteins, and DNA, producing progressively adverse changes that accumulate throughout the body and trigger a number of diseases. An ample outside source of antioxidants will assist in coping with this oxidative stress. While supplement studies have shown them to be mostly ineffective (and sometimes even harmful), the foods of the Mediterranean diet, rich in antioxidants such as vitamins A, C, and E, and thousands of phytochemicals, provide this important benefit.

Nowhere are vitamins, minerals, antioxidants, and phytochemicals more densely concentrated than in **fruits and vegetables**, an essential part of the Mediterranean diet. Studies show that, among their many benefits, they help protect against heart disease, stroke, and certain cancers, and a high intake is linked to lower body weight (in particular, the more vegetables you eat, the less body fat you're likely to have).

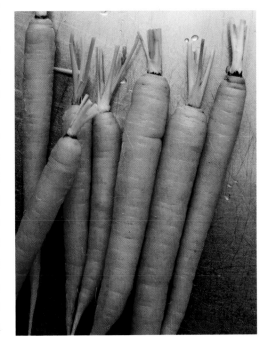

Eating plenty of one particular vegetable type— **legumes**—is such a distinctive and important component of the Mediterranean diet that I have separated it from the vegetable category in my book. Legumes include beans, lentils, peas, and soybeans. They are high in fiber, calcium, and iron, and are among the best protein sources in the plant kingdom. They also offer a rich supply of B vitamins, folic acid, minerals, antioxidants, and complex carbohydrates. The folic acid and vitamin B_6 in legumes help keep your heart healthy by breaking down homocysteine (an amino acid by-product from meat consumption that builds up in the blood and has been strongly linked with heart disease, stroke, and blood clots in the veins). Due to their filling high-fiber and protein contents, legumes also aid in weight loss and maintaining a healthy weight.

Mediterraneans also eat a lot of **fish**. Regularly eating fish has been associated with reduced risk of heart attack, sudden cardiac death, clotting-type stroke, and heart arrhythmias. The effect is mostly attributed to the omega-3 fats in oily, fatty fishes, though all fish have some. Of note, while omega-3 fats from plant sources also appear to benefit heart health, evidence points to a stronger effect from marine sources.

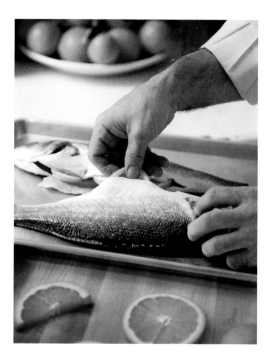

There is a theme that comes up over and over among the longest-lived people on earth: they eat a lot of **nuts**! Chock-full of healthy unsaturated fats, vitamins, minerals, antioxidants, and hunger-quelling protein, nuts appear to promote longevity across the Blue Zones (areas where people live measurably longer lives). Studies have been remarkably consistent in finding that nuts help prevent cardiovascular disease and heart attacks. For example, in a 1992 study of Seventh-day Adventists, those who consumed nuts at least five times a week had about half the risk of heart disease compared with those who didn't. This was true of men, women, vegetarians, and nonvegetarians, whether the nuts were roasted in oil or not. Studies have also reported possible benefits in reducing the risk of type 2 diabetes and some cancers.

Washing one's meal down with a glass of **wine** also seems to play a role in the healthy Mediterranean diet. Moderate alcohol consumption, in the absence of weight gain, has been associated with many health benefits, such as raising the good HDL cholesterol levels, raising factors that break down blood clots, reducing systemic inflammation, and improving insulin resistance. Consequently it is associated with less cardiovascular disease and diabetes. A lower risk of Alzheimer's and nonalcoholic fatty liver disease has also been observed. While recent studies suggest that it doesn't have to be wine (a glass of spirits or beer with your meal may have the same benefits), wine was the Mediterranean way when I was growing up. The lowest cardiovascular risk is seen among those who drink modestly several times a week, which was the pattern in my hometown of Castrofilippo as well. People would drink one to two glasses a night, mostly red wine, and would rarely overindulge.

The wide **variety of foods** eaten in the Mediterranean diet ensures consumption of a large assortment of important nutrients, as well as keeps any one particular toxin or pesticide that may be present in certain foods to a minimum. A study published in 1995 examining the connection between total dietary diversity (gauged by a score for the number of food groups consumed daily, be it from dairy, meat, grain, fruit, or vegetable) and subsequent overall mortality (including from cardiovascular disease and cancer) demonstrated an inverse relationship—so as variation in the diet went up, the chance of dying went down.

HEALTH EFFECTS

One of the most important influences diet can have upon health is simply by establishing **weight control**. Being overweight can damage every system in the body and is a risk factor for all of our most serious, debilitating diseases. The Mediterranean diet helps one maintain a healthy weight by providing complex carbohydrates, fiber, and protein to help you feel full and to slow digestion so you feel satisfied for longer. In addition, because the concentration is on fresh food, you're not eating commercially made products that are much higher in calories as well as designed to compel you to overeat and create irresistible cravings. It's also easy to follow because it doesn't involve an extreme diet makeover, and—as you'll see when you start trying recipes—it tastes so good!

One of the problems with weight gain is that surplus fat may settle within the torso, called **abdominal fat** (belly fat). This profile is particularly dangerous because the fat cells are not just layered under the skin where they are meant to be, but encircle vital internal organs. It's believed that once the ordinary fat cells reach capacity, fat cells set up camp in the abdomen, growing around the organs, heart, and vasculature. Substances released by the fat cells can then easily travel to the liver, where they can affect cholesterol levels. Abdominal fat is linked with higher bad LDL cholesterol, lower good HDL cholesterol, and is a major source of inflammatory compounds (more on that on the next page). The Mediterranean diet helps by promoting a healthy weight, and there is some evidence that it specifically helps reduce waist circumference, the customary measurement for abdominal fat.

You may have been hearing a lot about **inflammation** in the news these days, and you may be wondering what it is exactly and why it's so bad for you. Briefly, our immune system is designed to attack harmful substances and help repair damage in our bodies, and inflammation is the biological response mounted to deal with that. This is a good thing, obviously, and the process usually resolves on its own. White blood cells are sent to the site of the damage or foreign substance and a cascade of biochemical events gets the immune response going to mend you. If inflammation continues when it's not needed, however, it is destructive and primes us for disease.

When the inflammatory process goes on for too long, it causes "bystander" damage. The damaged tissue then keeps signaling the immune response for help, recruiting more and more white blood cells in a self-perpetuating loop, becoming chronic inflammation. Systemic inflammation involves the thin layer of cells that line the interior of blood vessels throughout the entire circulatory system. Atherosclerosis (plaque buildup within the walls of the arteries) involves a chronic inflammatory response of the blood vessels such as this; in fact, a fundamental role for inflammation has been established in all stages of the disease, from the very beginning to plaque and clot formation. Inflammation is also implicated in cancer, type 2 diabetes, Alzheimer's disease, and rheumatoid arthritis, among many other diseases. The Mediterranean diet reduces systemic inflammation, hence adherence is likely to improve or prevent any condition that is correlated with it.

The Mediterranean diet helps with **blood sugar regulation** by helping keep blood sugar levels appropriately low and even. This feature helps prevent diabetes, but not in the way you might think. Type 2 diabetes develops when the body stops responding to insulin, which results in harmful high blood sugar levels. Contrary to popular belief, diabetes is not caused by too much sugar in the diet. Rather, it's caused by too much of anything, which leads to excess pounds. The mechanism is still being clarified, but being overweight and lack of physical activity are responsible for nearly 95 percent of all diabetes cases in the United States, according to the Centers for Disease Control. The Mediterranean diet can help keep weight down as I discussed above. There is also some evidence that the anti-inflammatory effects of the diet help prevent diabetes. Preventing sugar levels

Losing Weight on the Mediterranean Diet

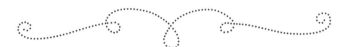

You might think that paying attention to food the way Italians do makes one obsess about it and leads to overeating, but it's quite the opposite. Instead of mindless, accidental consuming, it is conscientious obtaining, preparing, consuming, and appreciating, beginning from a very early age. This is a formula for recognizing the value of what's good and for rejecting adulterated, chemical-filled food products from the food industry. If you have pounds to lose, below are some useful suggestions to try.

- Protein-rich foods are the most filling, both during a meal and in between meals (followed, in order, by complex carbohydrates, simple carbohydrates, and, many might find surprising, fat). Good plant sources are nuts and legumes.
- Eat plenty of fiber-rich foods like legumes, whole grains, fruits, and vegetables, as fiber has no calories and is filling.
- Research indicates that replacing other types of fats with monounsaturated fats, especially olive oil, helps people lose weight.
- Change your snacks—out with processed foods and refined carbs.
- No more sugary drinks—they are a waste of calories, as they add no nutritional value, and studies show you don't register fullness drinking them as you would eating the same calories of solid food.
- Eat lots of fish—the protein in it is highly satiating, it's lower calorie than mammal meats, and its fats are good for you. Minimize other meats.
- Eat high volumes of low-calorie, healthy foods.
- Incorporate more physical activity into your days.
- Eat slowly and savor your food. The sensations will feel rewarding, and it will give you a chance to feel full and eat less.
- Control portion size by plating your meals and putting the rest away.

from spiking (by slowing digestion with fiber and complex carbohydrates) helps keep hunger in check as well.

Uncontrolled **high blood pressure** can lead to atherosclerosis, heart attack, stroke, aneurysm, heart failure, kidney disease, metabolic syndrome, trouble with memory or understanding, and vision loss caused by narrowed or torn blood vessels in the eyes. Although there is often not a firm identifiable cause, high blood pressure is strongly correlated with being overweight. Fatty tissue can increase resistance in blood vessels, which puts a strain on the heart; this increased mechanical strain can also cause damage to the vessels themselves, thus instigating the call for white blood cells and promoting systemic inflammation. The Mediterranean diet can counter this by helping you lose weight and reduce inflammation. The diet is also not high in salt; salt increases blood volume, which makes your heart work harder, and raises your blood pressure.

Blood lipids—meaning the fats in your blood as well as your blood **cholesterol** profile—have a large impact upon your health. The fats you eat influence your blood lipids the most. Polyunsaturated and monounsaturated fats are associated with high good HDL and low bad LDL levels—as are plant-based diets and fiber—all of which are hallmarks of the Mediterranean diet. In contrast, a diet high in saturated fat, trans fat, sugar, and/or refined carbohydrates results in an unfavorable lipid profile.

The Mediterranean diet provides copious antioxidants to help reduce **oxidation** in bodily processes. The many conditions in which oxidative damage is thought to play a significant role include atherosclerosis, all inflammatory conditions, certain cancers, clotting diseases (such as heart disease and stroke), AIDS, emphysema, the need for organ transplantation, gastric ulcers, hypertension and preeclampsia, neurological disorders (such as Alzheimer's disease, Parkinson's disease, muscular dystrophy), smoking-related diseases, and many others, as well as the process of aging.

Blood clotting is involved in the development of cardiovascular plaques to the formation of clots from ruptured plaques that clog arteries. It's been shown that substituting an unsaturated fat for a saturated fat reduces clot formation in vitro. Olive oil in particular has been demonstrated to have anticlotting properties, as do allium vegetables like garlic, onions, and leeks, all staples in the Mediterranean diet.

Calcium sources in the Mediterranean diet, as well as olive oil, contribute to **bone health**. Olive oil has been shown to help prevent osteoporosis in the elderly. The anti-inflammatory effects of the diet also help prevent conditions such as rheumatoid arthritis.

The Mediterranean diet also benefits the **nervous system** in terms of protecting neurons and preserving cognitive function. In many studies, it has been shown to be linked with a lower incidence of depression, which is generally attributed to its omega-3 fats. Its antioxidant and anti-inflammatory properties may be responsible for its protective effect upon degenerative brain diseases like Alzheimer's, Parkinson's, and Huntington's.

Finally, I'd like to revisit extra-virgin olive oil. Over the course of many studies and as many years, it has been shown to be a nutritional superstar. It . . .

- Reduces systemic inflammation
- Lowers bad LDL cholesterol
- Reduces LDL oxidation
- Raises good HDL cholesterol
- Improves blood vessel function
- Reduces blood clotting
- Promotes healthy blood pressure
- Prevents bone loss
- Facilitates weight control and lowers abdominal fat

Essentially, olive oil consumption addresses most of the health effects we have covered above. You can see why it's integral to the healthfulness of the Mediterranean diet—as well as to its flavor.

MEDITERRANEAN DIET SYNERGY

The theme of healthful eating overwhelmingly and consistently emphasizes the same pattern with the same group of foods: vegetables, fruits, legumes, nuts, seeds, and whole grains, with an emphasis on fish, skinless poultry, and plant foods as protein sources, and unsaturated plant oils such as olive oil. Modest amounts of low-fat dairy are usually included, but banished are trans fat, saturated fat, refined starches, and added sugar and salt. This diet should go along with regular physical activity as well as portion control to maintain a healthy weight.

So now we have put it all together: where the Mediterranean diet came from, how it makes us stronger, and how it can help us live a long, healthy life. In the next chapter, I will get into specific recommendations. Let the Mediterranean diet and lifestyle guide you and your family to a healthier, happier way of life.

EATING AND DRINKING:

The Fabulous 14

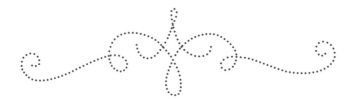

*Your well-being, and that of your family, is fundamentally based upon ordinary things done every day, throughout the day. In this section, I'll describe how to make daily healthy choices the Mediterranean way. I have distilled the essence of the diet into fourteen fabulous categories—see my recom-*mendations below with regard to fruits and vegetables, legumes, nuts, and seeds, whole grains, olive oil, healthy fats, protein, dairy and eggs, seafood, poultry and meat, wine, water, eating a wide variety of foods, and eating locally and seasonally, and you'll be ready to go!

THE MEDITERRANEAN DIET PYRAMID

Our Mediterranean diet pyramid reflects the idealized, life-prolonging diet of the southern Italians and residents of Crete in the 1950s and '60s, with some

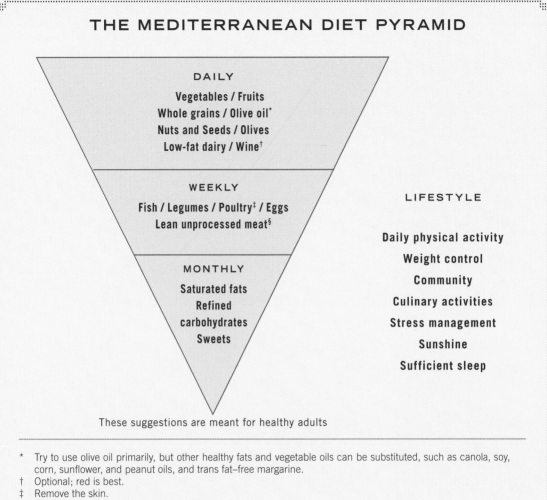

THE MEDITERRANEAN DIET PYRAMID

DAILY
Vegetables / Fruits
Whole grains / Olive oil*
Nuts and Seeds / Olives
Low-fat dairy / Wine†

WEEKLY
Fish / Legumes / Poultry‡ / Eggs
Lean unprocessed meat§

MONTHLY
Saturated fats
Refined
carbohydrates
Sweets

LIFESTYLE

Daily physical activity

Weight control

Community

Culinary activities

Stress management

Sunshine

Sufficient sleep

These suggestions are meant for healthy adults

* Try to use olive oil primarily, but other healthy fats and vegetable oils can be substituted, such as canola, soy, corn, sunflower, and peanut oils, and trans fat–free margarine.
† Optional; red is best.
‡ Remove the skin.
§ If red meat, try for organic, grass-fed beef.

adjustments in light of the latest nutritional research, and keeping in mind the contemporary weight control dilemma that affects so many. The considerable decline in modern daily physical activity levels alone makes our lives invariably different from theirs, and so we have to compensate for that.

The pyramid focuses on proportions of food servings within the diet as a whole to provide a sense of frequency for the various building blocks. It's not meant to be a rigid set of rules, as the amounts should vary based on your body size, your physical activity level, and your own tastes. It's a simple, flexible road map showing what to maximize and what to minimize.

WHAT TO EAT AND DRINK

Generally speaking, choose widely from the main categories of the Mediterranean diet (from meal to meal, and even within a meal). Choose healthy proportions, such as a plate consisting of half vegetables, a quarter whole grains or starchy vegetable (like sweet potato), and a quarter lean protein. Fill up on foods that are naturally low in calories like fruits and vegetables. Don't overdo it on the elements higher in calories such as olive oil, nuts, legumes, and pasta, and exercise overall portion control.

FRUITS AND VEGETABLES

HOW MUCH / HOW OFTEN: 5 to 8 servings every day (approximate serving size = 1 medium piece of fresh fruit, ½ cup chopped fruit, ¼ cup dried fruit, ½ cup cooked vegetables, 1 cup salad).

RECOMMENDATION: Fruits and vegetables are the mainstay of any healthy diet. Try to eat a generous portion of them at every meal. While you should strive to sample a broad array of fruits and vegetables, they're not all created equal. For example, cruciferous vegetables (like broccoli and cauliflower) and berries are the most densely nutritious vegetables and fruits.

Remember fruits and vegetables when choosing snacks and desserts as well! Don't forget dried fruits like prunes, dates, figs, raisins, and apricots. Note that fruits and vegetables have phytochemicals concentrated in their skins, so it's best to leave them on.

WATCH OUT FOR: Pesticides, which are used (and may be equally harmful) in both organic and commercial farming. Wash all produce under running water, including produce with peels that you'll cut through.

LEGUMES

HOW MUCH / HOW OFTEN: 3 to 4 servings per week (approximate serving size = ½ cup cooked).

RECOMMENDATION: Legumes are a terrific source of protein and are good alternatives to meat. They include beans, lentils, peas, garbanzo beans (chickpeas), navy beans, fava beans, alfalfa, clover, soybeans, peanuts, and carob.

WATCH OUT FOR: Legumes are relatively high in calories, so smaller portions are advised for those concerned with weight control.

WHY LEGUMES?

Legumes are grown and consumed quite frequently in the Mediterranean. Even though they're technically vegetables, I put them in a separate section in this book because many people overlook them, despite their importance in a healthy diet. For example, legumes are one of the plant kingdom's richest sources of protein. Protein is filling and so can help with weight loss. High-protein and low-carb plant-based diets significantly reduce the bad LDL cholesterol while promoting weight loss similar to that seen with the meat-based low-carb diets (which increase LDL). In fact, several studies have shown that deriving one's dietary protein from vegetables can reduce cholesterol levels to the same degree that statin drugs can! And while statins have little effect on raising the good HDL cholesterol, plant-based diets accomplish this as well. In my region of the Mediterranean, we ate some kind of legume every day.

NUTS AND SEEDS

HOW MUCH / HOW OFTEN: 4 to 5 servings per week (approximate serving size = 1 ounce [about ¼ cup] nuts or seeds, 1 tablespoon nut butter).

RECOMMENDATION: When you're feeling hungry in between meals, grab a handful of nuts—their protein is filling, and they're full of healthy fats, vitamins, minerals, and antioxidants. Add them to recipes or desserts, sprinkle them over a salad, or use them in place of meat in entrees. The best nuts and seeds are raw or roasted. If they're cooked in oil, check that it's a healthy oil (and note the increase in calories). A cooking oil and additive that's too sugary or salty can turn a healthy nut or seed snack into an unhealthy one. Some to try that have a great fat/nutrient profile: walnuts, almonds, cashews, pecans, Brazil nuts, pine nuts, pistachios, flaxseeds, chia seeds, sunflower seeds, pumpkin seeds, and sesame seeds.

WATCH OUT FOR: Though adding nuts to the diet in moderation has been shown not to cause weight gain, and in fact may help with weight loss by providing satiation, be careful not to overdo it. Their roughly 175 calories per ounce could add up quickly.

WHOLE GRAINS

HOW MUCH / HOW OFTEN: 3 servings a day (approximate serving size = 1 slice of bread, ¾ to 1 cup cereal, ½ cup cooked grains or pasta). While more servings used to be recommended, in light of pressing weight-maintenance concerns, the suggested number of servings has been reduced for the present time.

RECOMMENDATION: Eat minimally processed grains in preference to refined grains, which have had the healthy parts milled out of them. In addition to whole wheat products, try whole oats (steel-cut oats, rolled oats, old-fashioned oats), bran, barley, and brown rice. Semolina-based pasta (like De Cecco) is less refined and has higher protein and lower carbohydrate content than most other pastas, which makes it a low-glycemic index food (the glycemic index is a measurement showing how much a carbohydrate affects blood sugar—the lower the better).

WATCH OUT FOR: Refined grains (or "refined carbs") such as those in white bread, white rice, doughnuts, crackers, and instant oatmeal; also watch for high sodium levels in baked goods and rice mixes.

THE CARBOHYDRATE MYTH

Carbohydrates tend to get a bad rap these days because they are thought to be linked to weight gain and the obesity epidemic. While it's true that carbohydrates can be high in calories and you have to be cognizant of that, there is a wide range of dietary carbohydrate—some healthy, some not. The simplest carbohydrate is sugar, and that is what "high-carbohydrate diet" usually means in scientific studies. However, complex carbohydrates like those found in whole grains (and fruits and vegetables) are in a different category. The health benefits of diets rich in whole grains are conclusively established.

Minimally processed grains were an important staple in my family when I was a boy. My mother would make very dense, chewy, grainy bread every day. We always ate large portions because it was inexpensive and filling, and everyone could afford to make their own. We would eat it with everything—we'd dunk it in soups, and have it alongside salad, fish, or vegetables. Once we were in the US, my father valued good bread so much he would walk to a special bakery every day to get it, which I still do to this day.

The flour in Italy was not refined as it often is here. To find healthy bread in today's supermarket, make sure you are getting whole grain bread. Check the labels for ingredients, which are listed in descending order by weight. "Whole wheat flour" or "100% whole wheat flour" should be the first ingredient and the only flour listed. Terms like "wheat flour," "unbleached wheat flour," "multigrain," "enriched," or "stone-ground wheat flour" are just clever ways of saying refined white flour.

OLIVE OIL

HOW MUCH / HOW OFTEN: Varies widely, depending on one's weight, level of physical activity, age, and health, but generally try to include it in your diet every day.

RECOMMENDATION: Make olive oil your go-to oil when cooking. Drizzle fresh oil over salads and entrees, which is even better, since its nutrients degrade with heat and time. Use cold-pressed extra-virgin olive oil for optimal health benefits.

WATCH OUT FOR: Though following a Mediterranean diet relatively high in fat—mostly from olive oil—has not been shown to cause weight gain in studies, and in fact has been shown to be effective for weight loss, it is concentrated in calories (120 calories per tablespoon), so be careful not to overdo it.

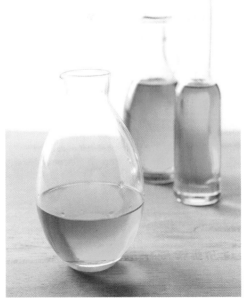

HEALTHY FATS AND OILS

HOW MUCH / HOW OFTEN: Varies widely depending on one's weight, level of physical activity, age, and health, but generally try to include some in your diet every day. Should be 25 to 40 percent of daily calories.

RECOMMENDATION: Get the majority of your fat from plant sources. Strive to incorporate plenty of monounsaturated fats (found in olive oil, canola oil, almonds, avocados, peanuts, and cashews) and omega-3 polyunsaturated fats from the sea (found in salmon, mackerel, tuna, anchovies, herring, trout, and sardines) and from plants (found in walnuts, flax, chia, and other seeds) into your diet. Include, but to a much lesser degree, omega-6 polyunsaturated fats (found in soybean, corn, sunflower, and safflower oils).

WATCH OUT FOR: Saturated fat, trans fats (partially hydrogenated fat), and excess omega-6 fats.

HEALTHY PROTEINS

HOW MUCH / HOW OFTEN: The amount of protein can be adjusted for an individual's age, health, level of physical activity, and weight control but, generally speaking, should not exceed 10 to 20 percent of daily calories.

RECOMMENDATION: Choose plant sources of protein as much as possible over animal proteins. Examples of good sources of protein are chickpeas (and hummus), lentils, black beans, pumpkin seeds, cashews, cauliflower, quinoa, pistachios, turnip greens, black-eyed peas, soy, avocado, kale, spinach, nut butters, chia seeds, and buckwheat.

WATCH OUT FOR: Protein from animal sources like meat and dairy, as it usually comes along with saturated fats, fewer nutrients, and a dearth of antioxidants. Excess protein can be harmful, and most people eat too much (adults require roughly 50 grams of protein per day).

DAIRY AND EGGS

HOW MUCH / HOW OFTEN: Eat a moderate amount of low-fat dairy (such as one serving a day) or a small amount of high-fat dairy. Four eggs or fewer per week has not been shown to contribute to heart disease. It is probably best not to exceed one egg per day.

RECOMMENDATION: More than one serving a day of low-fat dairy (such as 1 glass of milk or yogurt or 1½ ounces of hard cheese) appears to be unnecessary. There are better ways to get calcium and prevent osteoporosis, like exercising and consuming dark, leafy vegetables and legumes. Use cheese only as an accent to your dish, and choose low-fat versions of the dairy products you eat regularly.

WATCH OUT FOR: Dairy products high in fat, such as whole milk, cream, many cheeses, and ice cream. People with diabetes or heart disease should keep their egg-yolk consumption to three or fewer per week.

FISH AND SHELLFISH

HOW MUCH / HOW OFTEN: Aim for three to four servings of fish per week (especially fatty, oily fish). The FDA recommends that women who are pregnant (or planning to become so) or breastfeeding, as well as young children, should eat two to three servings of a variety of cooked seafood a week.

RECOMMENDATION: Eat a wide variety of seafood. If you are unable to eat fish, consult your doctor regarding fish oil supplements, especially if you have heart disease or are at high risk for it.

Ask the fish counter attendant what the freshest catch of the day is and form your meal around it. I encourage you to experiment with new types of seafood and to use the recipes found in "Fish and Other Seafood" (page 228) for inspiration on how to prepare them.

WATCH OUT FOR: Mercury content. Large predator fish tend to have accumulated the most, so consumption should not be excessive. Women planning to become pregnant or who are pregnant and young children should avoid king mackerel, swordfish, shark, and tilefish from the Gulf of Mexico for their mercury content (bigeye/ahi tuna is also quite high); albacore (white) tuna should be limited to 6 ounces per week.

SEEK OUT THESE *PESCE* (FISH) LOW IN MERCURY

Some people are nervous about eating fish because of environmental toxins, but in general, the health benefits outweigh these risks (except for pregnant women and young children). Methylmercury, polychlorinated biphenyls (PCBs), and dioxins, among others, are present in fresh waters and oceans, and in the animals that live in them as well. Risk from PCBs is normally small, however, and you can reduce it by removing the skin and fat.

The following fish are relatively low in mercury:

FRESH FISH: Smaller fish and shellfish such as herring, tilapia, shrimp, scallops, squid, crab, mussels, pollock, catfish, cod, salmon

CANNED FISH: Salmon, mackerel, light (yellowfin) tuna

SEAFOOD ALL-STARS (LOW IN MERCURY AND HIGH IN OMEGA-3S): Salmon (Alaskan king/Chinook, Atlantic, Coho, pink, and sockeye), arctic char, Atlantic mackerel, sardines, black cod, anchovies, oysters, rainbow (freshwater) trout, mussels, Pacific halibut, orata (bream), herring, squid, pollock, and canned salmon, mackerel, and tuna

POULTRY AND SMALL AMOUNTS OF LEAN MEAT

HOW MUCH / HOW OFTEN: Up to two meals per week, 3 ounces cooked (which is about the size of a deck of cards).

RECOMMENDATION: When I was growing up in Italy, most people in my area had meat only once every two weeks, if they could afford it. Limit meat as much as you can and try to use it as an accent rather than as the main attraction in a meal. Choose poultry over red meat. With red meat, choose unprocessed lean cuts such as rounds or loins from grass-fed livestock. When reducing meat, increasing legumes and nuts can satisfy your protein needs.

WATCH OUT FOR: Be sure to trim the skin off poultry; it's loaded with saturated fat. Don't smother lean meats with high-fat sauces and cheese. Avoid processed meats like bacon, sausages cured with nitrites, and lunch meats.

WINE

HOW MUCH / HOW OFTEN: Men may benefit from drinking one to two glasses of wine per day, and women up to one glass (one glass = 5 ounces).

RECOMMENDATION: This part of the Mediterranean diet is entirely optional, of course. Wine is best for your health if you drink it with a meal.

WATCH OUT FOR: Alcohol intake also has negative health effects. Those who are pregnant, are prone to addiction, are taking medication that adversely interacts with alcohol, have religious reasons to refrain, or have unpleasant reactions to alcohol should abstain.

WATER

HOW MUCH / HOW OFTEN: Drink at least eight glasses of water a day.

RECOMMENDATION: Drink for longevity—the longest-lived people on earth drink lots of water. Make drinking a glass of water a habit by doing it at certain times or places during the day.

The Fresher, the Better

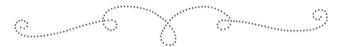

There is nothing better than eating fresh produce like a juicy summer peach, a crisp fall apple, or a just-picked sweet strawberry. In southern Italy, we used to have this luxury nearly all year round. We had a long summer, long spring (it started in February!), and the winters were very short, so throughout the year we always had something available. For a while there would be figs, then peaches—white and then yellow—then apricots, then cherries; every few weeks there was something new. Sometimes people harvested tomatoes twice a year. The taste was phenomenal.

Nowadays produce is shipped from all over, and it loses flavor as it loses moisture, which happens every step of the way—chilling, transport, and being held in warehouses all harm flavor.

In-season, local fruits and vegetables, on the other hand, don't have these flavor obstacles, and they're better for you, too. Produce picked and eaten at its peak generally has more vitamins, minerals, and antioxidants than foods harvested before they're ripe and that take a while to get to you. In fact, these fragile nutrients begin to break down as soon as the foods are picked.

WATCH OUT FOR: Both young children and the elderly are at increased risk of becoming seriously dehydrated and can't rely on thirst to signal they're not properly hydrated.

EAT A VARIETY OF FOODS

HOW MUCH / HOW OFTEN: Every meal, every day.

RECOMMENDATION: Maximize nutrients and minimize exposure to any one pesticide or toxin by choosing widely, especially among fruits, vegetables, and seafood. When it comes to produce, try to eat "colorfully" (blueberries, oranges, red apples, orange sweet potatoes, green zucchini, yellow squash, and so on); the colors are related to various phytochemicals and antioxidants, so you'll be sure to consume a cornucopia of nutrients.

WATCH OUT FOR: The winter season limits availability of fresh produce; these are times when things like frozen fruits—picked at their peak, washed thoroughly, and quickly frozen—can pack a more nutritious punch than fruit that has traveled halfway across the globe to your store.

EAT LOCALLY AND SEASONALLY

HOW MUCH / HOW OFTEN: Every meal, every day.

RECOMMENDATION: Local, in-season produce will taste better, be more nutritious, and save you money. Become familiar with what's in season in your area throughout the year. Seek out farmers' markets and you-pick farms. To find out what's harvested in your area, go to www.localharvest.org to find farmers' markets near you and seasonal produce guides.

WATCH OUT FOR: Though technically FDA-regulated, international produce may not have been subjected to much oversight in terms of pesticide monitoring, and only a small percentage is tested in the US.

TUTTI A TAVOLA: ALL TO THE TABLE, BABIES TO SENIORS

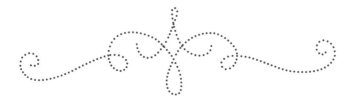

When Ancel Keys undertook his international studies to identify the communities that were the healthiest and longest-lived back in the 1950s and 1960s, he scrutinized only the grown-ups. Given that kids were eating essentially the same diet as their parents, clearly it was helping grow kids into healthy adults. As more studies on the Mediterranean diet were conducted over time, it became clear that the diet even benefited those who began it in their later years, helping them to recover from serious health conditions and to live longer overall. In this chapter, we'll examine the most pressing nutritional concerns at different stages of life, and learn how the Mediterranean diet can adapt and provide tasty, health-promoting options along the way.

Following each life-stage section, I've included a list of "Great Choices," which boils down all the nutritional information to foods that especially meet the needs of that period of life. While it's best for everyone to eat a wide variety of Mediterranean foods, these lists highlight foods that would be excellent to include in accordance with age or stage for optimum health, from babies to seniors.

CHILDREN

As more and more pediatric studies are conducted in modern times, our understanding of the specific benefits the Mediterranean diet offers children is growing. For example, kids following a Mediterranean-style diet have been found to be less likely to become overweight or obese (and the greater their adherence to it, the truer this is), or to develop respiratory problems such as asthma. They are also less likely to have attention deficit hyperactivity disorder (ADHD). Other possible benefits are better cognitive development, reduced allergies, and improved coordination. In addition, since atherosclerosis can begin forming in childhood and can take twenty-five years to become expressed as full-blown heart disease, it's never too early to begin protecting one's heart.

How we are fed and how we eat are essential contributors to our development—from infancy into toddlerhood and childhood, and on into the teenage years. This relatively short time period not only accounts for childhood health, but the path taken contributes to one's well-being for the many subsequent decades of adult life. How we come to feed ourselves can affect how long we will live, and how happy, contented, and pain-free that life will be. Let's look at what a healthy diet is at each stage of childhood and how to support this time of rapid growth and development in an optimal way.

NEWBORN THROUGH FOUR MONTHS

The benefits of breastfeeding are well established (and for premature infants—those born prior to thirty-seven weeks—even more so). With the exception of vitamin D, which is generally suggested as a supplement to be taken by the mother, breast milk is fully adequate for the newborn, and its composition changes in sync with the baby's nutritional and growth needs. It is generally recommended to breastfeed exclusively for the first six months if possible. Among the many advantages to this is that it establishes a palate for the baby, who experiences through the breast milk the variety of flavors of food consumed by the mother. Breast-fed infants are less picky and more willing to try new foods later, which means they usually eat more fruits and vegetables in childhood. A full Mediterranean diet will provide healthy fats and vital nutrients to nourish a nursing mother and her developing infant.

Keep These Off Baby's Menu for the First Year

- Chocolate
- Egg whites
- Nuts
- Cow's milk
- Honey[*]

[*] Honey can contain botulism spores that can make young babies sick; the spores can only be killed by extremely high heat obtained in something like a pressure canner, so regular cooking is still risky.

HOW THE MEDITERRANEAN DIET HELPS THE NURSING MOTHER

- The fats a mother eats are reflected in her milk supply, so keep them Mediterranean healthy.
- Omega-3 fats, DHA in particular (which in nature is found in fatty fish like salmon, mackerel, and anchovies), have been found to be particularly beneficial to a baby's cognitive development.[*] They also may reduce postpartum depression in the mother.
- Many vitamins in the mother's diet, as well as calcium, are expressed in her breast milk.

GREAT CHOICES FOR MOM FOR THIS TIME OF LIFE: **Salmon, canned light tuna, oranges, sweet potatoes, carrots, ricotta cheese, green leafy vegetables, spinach,**

[*] While studies have not shown an ill effect related to seafood with mercury, the FDA recommends that nursing mothers, to be prudent, should abstain from the same fish that pregnant women and young children should avoid: larger predator fatty fish such as swordfish, tilefish from the Gulf of Mexico, king mackerel, and shark.

broccoli and broccoli rabe, fortified cereals, legumes, asparagus, enriched pasta, cantaloupe, eggs.

FIVE MONTHS THROUGH ONE YEAR

As the baby begins solid foods, we switch from recommendations for what the mother should eat to what is best for the baby.

During the first year of a child's life, the rate of growth and development is more rapid than at any other period in the life cycle. While a mother's milk can perfectly support this phase for the first months of life, at somewhere around five to six months, babies will begin to require more to sustain them: it will be time to begin their journey on solid foods.

Commercial baby foods are often used because of their sanitation and convenience; however, they are not a necessity, and I recommend limiting them. Instead, parents can prepare baby foods at home using a blender or food processor or by mashing well with a fork to create a soupy consistency. When you do it yourself, you can be assured that your child is getting a wide variety of fresh, nutritious foods without any harmful additives. If you are eating a healthy Mediterranean diet yourself, as you should be, you will already have these foods at home, so it can truly be a diet for the family from the very beginning.

Keep in mind that because infants are growing so rapidly, their **protein** requirements are greater relative to their size. Infants also require a higher **fat** intake, because fats provide energy to the developing liver, brain, and muscles, including the heart. Infants use fat more regularly for generating energy. However, do not add any salt, sugar, or butter, even if the food tastes bland to you, because babies don't miss it.

A ROUGH GUIDE TO BEGINNING SOLIDS

Add only one new food at a time over the course of two to three days in order to determine whether any allergic reactions arise. By nine months, a baby is are ready for finger food, and by the baby's first birthday, solid foods can make up around 50 percent of nutrition. Gradually increase variety and texture. Baby's job is to eat as much as desired at each mealtime, according to need, mood, capability, and preference. Allow for exploration and experimentation. Teach your child that food is to be enjoyed.

The importance of offering your child a wide variety of tastes in the early solid-food phase cannot be overstated. There is reason to believe that early food exposures may play an important role in establishing lifelong preferences. Studies of infants aged four to seven months showed that acceptance of new foods was more rapid at that time than after the first year of life. Aside from an innate fondness for the taste of sweet, food preferences of infants are largely learned. They like what is familiar to them—in other words, whatever becomes familiar, they come to like, which makes sense from a survival perspective.

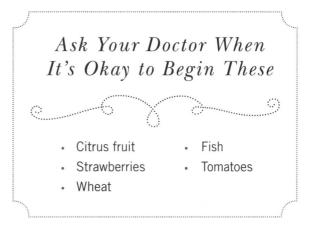

Ask Your Doctor When It's Okay to Begin These

- Citrus fruit
- Strawberries
- Wheat
- Fish
- Tomatoes

Offering a variety of food promotes progress in other ways as well. Feeding plays a role in the infant's developmental and early learning needs by providing a variety of tastes, colors, temperatures, and textures. The feeding experience itself offers valuable physical contact and visual, auditory, and social interaction.

AVOID

- FRUIT JUICE Babies under six months of age should not be given fruit juice, and it should be limited after that, especially until one year of age (and only 100 percent pasteurized fruit juice if store-bought). Juice fills the appetite, so drinking too much displaces other more nutritious foods, and it can lead to obesity. It's recommended that you dilute it by adding 10 parts water to 1 part juice.
- NITRATES Infants are the age group most likely to be affected by nitrates. Because of this, babies under the age of six months should be given limited quantities of vegetables like spinach and beets and should eat limited quantities of food that contain additives (like cheese and cured meats).
- TRANS FATS Surprisingly, baby foods and biscuits may contain trans fats. Read the labels and avoid them.

- PESTICIDES Organophosphates are among the most worrisome pesticides, and one of the most widely utilized. The developing nervous system, including the brain, of fetuses and young children is particularly at risk. The following produce consistently carries the highest levels of pesticides, even after home washing and peeling: peaches, apples, bell peppers, celery, nectarines, strawberries, cherries, pears, imported grapes, spinach, lettuce, and potatoes. See page 87 for how to best clean produce.
- SALT Salty foods are a learned preference and should be avoided from the very beginning so kids don't develop a taste for them. Salt should never be added to baby food. Avoid using processed foods, especially those made for adults such as cooking sauces, as these can be high in added salt.

GREAT CHOICES FOR THIS TIME OF LIFE: Iron-fortified cereal, bananas, pears, applesauce, carrots, sweet potatoes, winter squash, avocados, meat, tofu, peas, eggs, cheese, yogurt, finger foods like small pasta pieces.

Yogurt:
One of the Oldest Health Foods

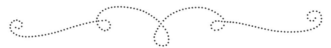

The culturing process with live bacteria makes yogurt ultra-digestible. Babies can eat it even before they're old enough to digest plain cow's milk. Yogurt is also packed with vitamins and nutrients, improves gastrointestinal function, boosts immunity, and may help protect against carcinogens and certain diseases. Just be sure to get yogurt with live cultures. An LAC label, for "Live & Active Cultures," will assure this; the line "made with live cultures" isn't sufficient—that could mean the yogurt was pasteurized later.

TODDLERS (TWO THROUGH THREE YEARS)

Although children's growth rate begins to slow down after the first year of life, they continue to need enough calories and essential nutrients to maintain growth and activity levels. Their preferences may change from day to day. Toddlers and preschoolers may go through a phase where they are willing to eat only a limited number of what used to be their favorite foods. If you give in to this, however, and serve the same foods over and over, you are further strengthening their preferences for these foods and narrowing the range of foods they're likely to eat. Instead, adults should decide when food will be offered and provide a consistent schedule, serve a variety of nutritious foods from which the child can choose, and set a good example by also eating an array of healthy foods. Given that toddlers are highly attuned to taste, texture, and temperature, slight adjustments may be able to turn their preferences around. As with infants, be patient, and don't force them to eat more food than they want or need.

These first few years are formative, so teach your child to enjoy the flavor of fresh food. If Baby begins with solid food from a jar, Baby concludes that this is what food is supposed to taste like. Packaged and fast foods will taste like the norm. On the other hand, if Baby and Toddler eat only homemade, freshly prepared, unsalted, unsweetened foods, this is the standard to which they will compare all other foods.

Because toddlers have a critical need for nutrients but a small stomach size (it's only about the size of their fist), they must eat frequently. It's best to serve a smaller portion of the food you expect them to eat so they aren't visually overwhelmed, and so they are allotted some control in asking for more. Don't let toddlers graze all day on snacks, or they'll never work up an appetite for the nutritious foods you'd like them to eat. A typical eating pattern should include a snack between breakfast and lunch, and between lunch and dinner, as well as a bedtime snack if needed.

THE GROWING YEARS

From birth through adolescence, children are growing and require proper nutrition to support their development. Periods of height increase are followed by brief plateaus and then by periods of weight gain. Children's appetite and nutrient needs are greatest during the growth phases. Providing a nutritious diet is crucial, as failure to meet nutrient needs for growth may result not only in a smaller stature but also in decreased resistance to illness and disease, lack of energy, and delays in physical and mental development.

Children require an adequate amount of protein, fat, carbohydrates, vitamins, minerals, and fluids. Below I'll discuss special concerns for each (see the table in the Appendix, page 305, for good food sources).

Carbohydrates should be a child's primary source of energy, because they are a concentrated source of energy and are easily digestible. About half of a child's calories should come from carbohydrates, especially complex carbohydrates in the form of fresh fruits, vegetables, starches, and whole grains.

Children's need for **protein** relative to their size remains very high from infancy through the preschool years, due to their continued rapid growth. Meat, milk, and eggs offer complete proteins, with all of the essential amino acids a body requires, whereas plant sources of protein (such as grains, legumes, and nuts) are incomplete, so a variety need to be eaten to achieve all of the required amino acids.

Fat is an essential nutrient for young children and is required for normal growth and development. It also provides the most concentrated source of energy. There should be no dietary fat restriction for children under two years of age unless they have a family history of obesity, heart disease, or diabetes. After that, fat intake in the diet should be 30 to 35 percent of daily calories for two- to three-year-olds, and 25 to 30 percent for four- to eighteen-year-olds. As found in the Mediterranean diet, it appears that **monounsaturated and polyunsaturated fats** are the best fats for children.

Because of their rapid growth, infants and young children require some **vitamins** in greater amounts relative to their body weight as compared with adults (such as **vitamins A, D, C, B$_6$, B$_{12}$, and folic acid**). While sometimes supportive, a multivitamin supplement is not a substitute for a healthy diet. Vitamin pills do not supply protein, fiber, essential fatty acids, and substances as yet unidentified in foods that are vital to good health.

Minerals help to regulate body functions and build tissue. **Calcium** and **phosphorus** are the major minerals required for healthy bone and teeth formation. **Iron** is essential for forming healthy blood, and normal growth depends on a healthy blood supply to nourish an increasing number of cells. Studies of children's nutritional status have repeatedly identified calcium and iron intakes to be inadequate.

Children need plenty of **water** for hydration, digestion, excretion, and growth. They experience more rapid water loss through evaporation and dehydration than do adults. Consequently, when children are busy or engaged in vigorous physical activity, they may need reminders to drink water.

GREAT CHOICES FOR THIS TIME OF LIFE: Sweet potatoes, carrots, green leafy vegetables, ricotta cheese, yogurt, cantaloupe, apricots, fish, edamame, oranges, bananas, avocados, spinach, canned tuna, broccoli, asparagus, eggs, enriched pasta, beans, peas, milk, whole grains.

YOUNG CHILDREN (FOUR THROUGH EIGHT YEARS)

In the preschool years (ages four to five), growth continues somewhat slowly compared with infancy, and children have a relatively small appetite and food intake. You may notice that appetite increases in advance of a growth spurt, causing children to add some weight that will be used for the upcoming sprout in height. Consequently, as with toddlers, their appetites can be quite variable.

Children do *not* have inborn mechanisms that direct them to select and consume a well-balanced diet. Most have preferences for foods that are high in calories with high levels of sugar and fat. Children will thus only learn healthful eating habits from their caregivers.

In middle childhood (age five to preadolescence), children continue to grow at a steady rate. Good nutrition continues to play an important role, ensuring that children reach their full potential for growth, development, and health.

Parents and older siblings still have the most influence on a child's attitudes toward food during this time, though peers and advertising begin to compete and may have some sway on children's wishes. Families should try to eat meals together. During this time, healthy eating habits are modeled and strengthened, and conversation and manners are practiced and absorbed. Make an effort for mealtimes to be a positive, bonding time for everyone.

NUTRITIONAL NEEDS

Youth and young adulthood is the period when bones build up to their peak strength. Helping children lead a bone-healthy lifestyle—with exercise, adequate **calcium,** and adequate **vitamin D** for calcium absorption—can help them keep strong bones through all their adult years. Milk is a key source of calcium and vitamin D, protein, and other essential micronutrients for kids. The ideal amount of milk and calcium isn't exactly clear, but two glasses per day appears to be sufficient. For children two years and older, instead of whole milk, go for low-fat and skim because they contain much less saturated fat than reduced-fat or whole milk.

In addition to calcium, other nutrients it's important to get enough of, and that sometimes fall short, are **iron, fiber, zinc,** and **protein** (see my table in the Appendix, page 305, for food sources). Meeting children's protein requirements ensures that there is protein enough to spare for tissue repair and growth.

AVOID

- FRUIT JUICE Fruit juice is loaded with sugar, sometimes even more so than soda. One study showed that the risk of obesity in children was increased by 60 percent for each daily serving of a sugar-sweetened beverage, which includes fruit juice. Excess fruit juice consumption by preschool-aged children is also associated with short stature.
- SODA Soda has all the problems of fruit juice, above, and then some. Its carbonation also inhibits phosphorus absorption, which is important for growth.
- SALT Once your little ones are eating the same foods as the rest of the family it is important to continue not adding any salt to their food. It is at this point that children's salt intake tends to increase dramatically. Homemade meals cooked using fresh ingredients

are naturally lower in salt than convenience meals and processed food.

- PROCESSED MEAT Processed meats—like bacon, ham, hot dogs, and deli meat—have been found to be less healthy than unprocessed red meat (likely due to the nitrites and nitrosamines they're cured with). It appears that they are especially harmful to children and have been linked to leukemia.
- ARTIFICIAL FOOD COLORINGS These contribute to hyperactivity in some children, and some food dyes have cancer risks.

GREAT CHOICES FOR THIS TIME OF LIFE: Beans, iron-fortified cereal, dried fruits, peas, whole grains like oats and barley, apples, pears, raspberries, bananas, oranges, strawberries, broccoli, corn, beans, oats, barley, eggs, edamame, yogurt, milk, cheese, kale.

THE OLDER CHILD (NINE THROUGH EIGHTEEN YEARS)

Preadolescence and adolescence span a time of profound biological, emotional, social, and cognitive changes during which children develop into adults. The dramatic physical growth and development they experience significantly increases their need for energy, protein, vitamins, and minerals. At the same time, the struggle for independence that characterizes this period often leads to health-compromising eating behaviors, such as excessive or fad dieting, meal skipping, use of supplements, and making unhealthy food choices when away from parental observation.

Too often teens hear the message that they should eat what they don't like because it's good for them. Instead, focus on the immediate, socially relevant issues that are important to them, such as their physical appearance, energy level, sports performance, and the environmental or moral aspects of food. Even though they need to be aware of the long-term risks of an unhealthy diet, focusing on tangible present benefits will more likely appeal to them and result in better nutritional choices.

These years may be challenging in terms of getting kids to eat healthfully.

But don't give up, because it's also a time when they need good-quality nutrients. For example, undernutrition and underweight can result in short stature as an adult. Because this is a time when kids are deciding who they want to be, the strength of one's family can provide a foundation and guide for the teenager. The search for personal identity can lead to positive behaviors such as the adoption of healthful eating practices, participation in competitive sports, and an overall interest in developing a healthy lifestyle. Be patient, continue to make family time a priority in your home, continue with your message of why nutrition matters, and continue to be a good role model.

The Mediterranean diet is an excellent means of achieving nutrient needs for the growing teen. Refer to my table in the Appendix (page 305) for good food sources for the nutrients.

NUTRITIONAL NEEDS

Increases in muscle, bone, and body fat that occur during puberty result in high caloric and nutrient needs exceeding those at any other point in life (specific requirements are influenced by activity level, metabolic rate, and growth phase).

The estimated **protein** need for teens is slightly higher than for adults. Protein requirements are highest (depending on growth patterns) for females aged eleven to fourteen years and males fifteen to eighteen, when growth is at its peak. When protein intake is inadequate during this period, reduction in height, delay in sexual maturation, and reduced lean body mass development may be seen. Vegetarians must pay close attention to achieving sufficient protein levels.

Getting enough **calcium** during adolescence is crucial to physical growth and development, as calcium is the main constituent of bones. Adequate intake is particularly important for athletes, especially girls, who have an increased risk of bone fracture. About half of peak bone mass is accumulated during adolescence, so calcium is of great importance for building dense bones and thus reducing the lifetime risk of fractures and osteoporosis. The recommended daily amount of calcium for nine- to eighteen-year-olds is 1,200 milligrams. Data suggest that female teens often consume far less than this.

Vitamin D is also essential for bone formation, thus an adequate amount is critical during adolescence. Since it is synthesized in the skin with direct sun exposure, those who do not get much sun may be deficient (as well as dark-skinned individuals, whose skin produces less). Vitamin D insufficiency is common among teens. The American Academy of Pediatrics recommends that all teens who do not consume at least 400 IU per day through dietary sources should receive a 400 IU supplement.

Even for teenagers, **sugar** affects cardiovascular health. A 2011 study showed that the more sugar teens consumed, the greater their cardiovascular risk factors were (their good HDL cholesterol dropped, their bad LDL cholesterol rose, and their triglycerides rose).

The rapid rate of vertical growth, increase in blood volume, and, for girls, the onset of menstruation increase teens' need for **iron**. While full-blown anemia is not common, iron deficiency among teens is prevalent, particularly among girls, thus iron should be a focus in teen nutrition. The required amount is based on sexual maturation level.

Folate is integral to protein synthesis. Evidence indicates that folate insufficiency is common among teens. Teens who skip breakfast or do not commonly consume orange juice and ready-to-eat fortified cereals are at an increased risk for having low folate levels.

Physical activity plays a role in bone development during adolescence. Participation in weight-bearing activities (strength training) leads to increased bone density in adulthood as compared to sedentary teens. For teenagers who are involved in sports with a high level of physical activity, calorie, protein, fluid, and select vitamin and mineral needs increase but vary widely. When the main source of protein is plant-based, additional protein may be needed.

The prevalence of **teens who are overweight** has nearly tripled in the past twenty-five years. This appears to be related to inadequate levels of physical activity, high-calorie diets, and excess consumption of sweetened beverages. Studies show that keeping to the Mediterranean diet will help your teen avoid becoming overweight. As at any age, teenagers will eat what's available and convenient, so keep healthy choices stocked. See my list of Tasty Mediterranean-Approved Snacks (pages 78–79), and avoid snacks with ingredients from my "What Not to Eat" list (page 56).

GREAT CHOICES FOR THIS TIME OF LIFE: Milk, cheese, yogurt, canned salmon, broccoli, kale, turnips, edamame, eggs, seafood, nuts and seeds, beans, peas, lentils, dried fruits, spinach, asparagus, cantaloupe, enriched pasta, meat.

ADULTS

Unless otherwise specified, the recommendations throughout my book are meant for adults. Here I'll briefly address a few special concerns: young adulthood, pregnancy, middle age, and menopause.

YOUNG ADULTHOOD

Young adulthood, a time of transition from the childhood home to college or an independent life, is a time full of change. Meal preparation, food and beverage availability, metabolic rate, and physical activity levels may suddenly be vastly different. Often weight gain is a result.

As far as nutritional recommendations during this life stage, embrace the full recommendations of the Mediterranean diet and lifestyle. This will give you energy, strength, and the best armor available to prevent you from becoming overweight and from developing future health problems.

GREAT CHOICES FOR THIS TIME OF LIFE: On-the-go snacks such as nuts, seeds, low-fat yogurt, chilled shrimp, hard-boiled eggs, cheese, banana, apple, orange, grapes, cherry tomatoes, trail mix, canned tuna in oil, dried fruits like apricots, figs, and raisins.

PREGNANCY

A pregnant woman should concentrate on increasing her nutrient intake, rather than her caloric intake, particularly in the first and second trimesters. She should bear in mind that the flavors she eats during pregnancy may be passed on as preferences to her unborn child. Hence, a diet that includes fruits, vegetables, and other healthy foods—especially if she continues to eat them during the newborn/breastfeeding stage—may be accepted more readily when her baby begins eating solid foods. These preferences may even last a lifetime.

Complete nutritional guidance on pre-pregnancy, pregnancy, and post-pregnancy/lactation is beyond the scope of this book, but some general recommendations include:

- Concentrate on **diet quality**, rather than quantity.
- Nutrients for which there are increased requirements during pregnancy include **folate**, **iron**, **vitamin B$_{12}$**, and **iodine**.
- The recommended intake of **calcium** does not specifically increase during pregnancy, but it's very important that pregnant women meet their calcium requirements.
- **Omega-3 fats** are extremely important for development in the growing fetus. The omega-3 fats found in seafood in particular have been shown to help neural development in the unborn child. Be careful with foods that are more likely to contain mercury, though. See page 92 for a list of seafood that maximizes omega-3s while minimizing mercury.

GREAT CHOICES FOR THIS TIME OF LIFE: Lentils and other legumes, broccoli, asparagus, enriched pasta, cantaloupe, eggs, fortified cereals, dried fruits, green leafy vegetables, salmon and other seafood (including canned tuna), iodized salt, yogurt, milk, cheese.

MIDDLE AGE

THE FORTIES

The forties are a period of active family responsibilities as well as expanding work and professional roles. Managing schedules and meals may become a challenge (see my lists of tips for saving time and money on pages 66 and 67). This may be a time of beginning to recognize one's mortality. While the forties mark a subtle decrease in bodily function, dietary and lifestyle recommendations remain the same as in earlier adulthood, and a healthy approach can vastly slow down the clock.

THE FIFTIES AND SIXTIES

For most adults over fifty, work, career, and family continue to be priorities. However, health concerns are frequently added to the picture. Health shortcuts taken over the years may be backfiring and are beginning to beget consequences. Managing risk factors to prevent disease or dealing with a disease or condition may now be an added responsibility.

In this life stage, as bodily functions slightly decline, the benefits of healthy eating include increased mental acuteness, resistance to illness and disease, higher energy levels, faster recuperation times, and better management of chronic health problems. As we age, eating well can also be a key component to having a positive outlook and staying emotionally balanced. As always, healthy eating doesn't have to be about dieting and sacrifice. Whatever your age, eating well should be all about fresh, colorful food, creativity in the kitchen, and eating with friends and people you love.

NUTRITIONAL NEEDS IN MIDDLE AGE

- **Calories**—You need fewer calories every decade. We move around less, we have less muscle, and our metabolic rate goes down.
- **Vitamin B_{12}**—After age fifty, your body's ability to absorb the B_{12} vitamin often fades, because you don't have as much stomach acid, which is needed to break B_{12} down from food sources.
- **Vitamin D**—Aging skin is less able than younger skin to change sunlight to vitamin D. That, in turn, affects the body's ability to absorb calcium. You need both vitamin D and calcium to prevent bone loss.

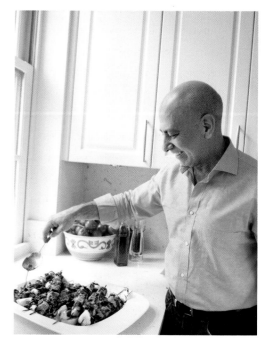

- **Potassium**—Blood pressure tends to rise as we age. To combat this problem and lower stroke and heart attack risk, you should eat less sodium and more potassium.
- **Salt**—Since salt and sodium contribute to the ascent of blood pressure as one gets older, they should be minimized. Get more potassium to counter the effects of salt.
- **Calcium**—Calcium is good for your bones and is found in dairy products and other

foods. Adults should get 1,000 milligrams a day; for women over fifty and men over seventy, that rises to 1,200 milligrams.

- **Lutein**—To save your eyes from age-related macular degeneration or cataracts, start upping your intake of lutein during middle age. According to some research, this nutrient may also help fend off cognitive decline.
- **Fiber**—Fiber needs increase as you get older. Fiber intake is key for normal bowel function and may lower the risk of gastrointestinal inflammation and disease. Plus, it can lower cholesterol and blunt the rise in blood sugar that occurs after eating.

GREAT CHOICES FOR THIS TIME OF LIFE: Spinach, broccoli, oranges, potatoes with skin, milk, fortified cereals, bananas, apples, pears, green leafy vegetables, grapes, whole grains, yogurt, radicchio, egg yolks.

MENOPAUSE

The decline of estrogen production in women begins in perimenopause (which varies widely but typically starts in the mid-forties) and continues through menopause. Due largely to these changes in estrogen, menopause is associated with an increase in abdominal fat, a significant increase in the risk of cardiovascular disease, and accelerated bone loss. Recommendations for menopausal women include:

- **Eat foods rich in calcium**, such as milk, or, if necessary, take calcium supplements as prescribed by a doctor.
- **Vitamin D** in adequate amounts will facilitate calcium absorption.
- **Weight-bearing exercises** such as walking or weight training will help strengthen bones and maintain a healthy body weight.
- **A high-fiber, low-fat, and low-salt diet** high in phytoestrogens has been found to reduce many symptoms of menopause, such as hot flashes. The Mediterranean diet has specifically been shown to reduce symptoms.

- **Olive oil** may also help strengthen bones—yet another reason to go Mediterranean at this stage of life.
- **Eating a well-balanced Mediterranean diet** will help prevent menopausal weight gain.

GREAT CHOICES FOR THIS TIME OF LIFE: Fennel, chickpeas, lentils, apples, pears, whole grains, edamame and other soy products, yogurt, green leafy vegetables, fish, broccoli, collard greens, turnips.

SENIORS: AGE SIXTY AND BEYOND

What counts as old depends on who's counting—the government has one definition; in your mind there is perhaps another. For my purposes, when I refer to older adults, seniors, or the elderly, I am referring to ages sixty and over, since for most people, nutritional needs shift from general adult and middle-age needs at this time. For example, daily calorie need declines from early adulthood on, about 100 calories less per decade to compensate for reduced physical activity and basal metabolic rate. Post-menopause is also accompanied by hormonal changes that often cause women to gain weight, and they gain it in the abdominal region, which is the riskiest place to carry fat. Organ function declines, chewing and swallowing may become more difficult, and gastrointestinal problems such as constipation and diverticulitis are common.

When we review studies about people who have followed the Mediterranean diet in their later years, the overriding message is that it's never too late to get healthier and add on years with the Mediterranean diet. Here are some of the specific benefits:

Cardiovascular health—Studies with elderly subjects show that the Mediterranean diet exerts its effects by reducing risk factors for cardiovascular disease, as well as by lessening the severity of the disease if one is already afflicted. Over and over, studies show that older adults have lower incidences of cardiac events like heart attacks, shorter hospitalization times, better outcomes, and fewer recurrences the more they adopt a Mediterranean-style diet.

Cancer—Data from many studies show the Mediterranean diet imparts a protective effect for certain cancers among older people.

Mental health—Observing the Mediterranean diet has been shown to reduce the incidence of Alzheimer's disease, increase cognitive performance among the elderly, and lower the occurrence of depression.

Musculoskeletal health—Studies have shown that there are very low rates of osteoporosis and osteoporosis-related fractures in the Mediterranean Basin, the lowest in the European Union. Adherence to a traditional Mediterranean diet has been associated with higher bone mineral density and lower fracture risk. A recent study suggests that olive oil consumption may be a factor. The Mediterranean diet has also been shown to improve rheumatoid arthritis.

Eye health—A Mediterranean diet reduces the risk of the most common cause of poor eyesight in older people. In an Australian study it was demonstrated that people who consume at least 100 ml (about 3½ ounces) of olive oil a week are almost 50 percent less likely to develop macular degeneration than those who consume less than 1 ml per week.

Life span—Studies have shown that the more faithfully people follow the Mediterranean diet, the longer they live. For example, in a large study of men aged seventy to ninety who followed the diet for ten years, adherence to the Mediterranean diet and healthful lifestyle was associated with a 50 percent lower rate of death from all causes. Interestingly, this protective effect upon mortality has been shown to be even stronger for individuals older than 55 years of age compared with younger people.

As people age, the role of nutrition changes somewhat. Rather than thinking of diet as a way to reduce the risk of future disease, in addition to keeping weight in check, it begins to affect everyday wellness and quality of life more than ever before. Wellness means having the energy and ability to comfortably do the things one wants to do and to feel in control of one's life, for as long as possible. In other words, as our bodies begin to naturally deteriorate, good nutrition can add life to years, as well as years to life. In general, older adults should:

- **Eat foods packed with nutrients.**
- **Choose fiber-rich foods often.**

- **Drink lots of water** and other beverages low in sugar.
- **Eat fortified foods or take supplements to get sufficient vitamins D and B$_{12}$.**
- **Eat healthy fats** such as olive oil and the fats found in fish and nuts.
- **Eat healthy carbohydrates** (like whole grains) to maintain a lower weight, rest the pancreas (the insulin-pumping organ whose functioning goes awry in diabetes), help smooth gastrointestinal function, and maximize the intake of healthy nutrients per calories consumed.
- **Be sure to get enough protein**, as older adults are prone to insufficient protein intake, leading to weakened muscles and bones, and a diminished immune system and delay wound healing.
- **Limit sweets** to decrease empty calories.

NUTRITIONAL NEEDS

Health can be maximized at this stage of life with the Mediterranean diet. In general, older adults eat less, so they require foods denser in nutrients. Certain nutrients require attention due to low dietary intake and changes in absorption and metabolism. The most common nutrient concerns are getting too little vitamins D, B$_{12}$, E, and K, folate, calcium, magnesium, and potassium, and getting too much vitamin A and iron. See below for more detail, and refer to page 305 for good food sources.

Vitamin D is of particular concern, as many older adults are deficient, and it's necessary for optimal calcium absorption to keep bones from becoming brittle. Seniors' ability to manufacture it in the skin goes way down, plus they may not be outside in the sun as much to activate its production, and they may take medications that interfere with its metabolization.

Vitamin A may be too high in many older adults, which can cause liver damage. Excess vitamin A can cause hair loss, dry skin, nausea, irritability, blurred vision, and/or weakness. Be aware of foods that are rich in vitamin A, like carrots and sweet potatoes. Like vitamin A, **iron** is stored more readily in the old than in the young. Excess iron contributes to oxidation, thus increased antioxidant exposure is helpful to deal with the overload. Watch consumption of iron-rich foods like fortified cereals and red meat, which can contribute too much iron.

On Supplements

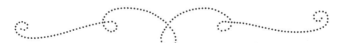

While in general it's advisable to consume your vitamins and minerals through healthy foods, later in life, supplements may be beneficial in certain cases. You should consult your doctor for this, as it will depend on your personal diet, health conditions, health risks, and any medications you're taking.

Vitamin C is recommended because it may help protect against bone loss, serves as an antioxidant, and increases iron absorption if needed.

A common theme among the nutrients is that the balance becomes more delicate—one is more vulnerable to both excess and inadequacy, and either can easily cause health problems. For example, calcium absorption declines with age, but too much will cause kidney stones. Medications are also more common later in life and affect how the body uses nutrients. Thus, a healthy diet, and awareness of one's nutritional status, are more important than ever before.

GREAT CHOICES FOR THIS TIME OF LIFE: Sunshine, fish, soy, salmon, canned tuna, nuts and seeds, whole grains, green leafy vegetables, yogurt, cheese, bananas, oranges, cantaloupe, raisins, legumes, winter squash, spinach, broccoli, molasses, dark chocolate, olive oil, Brussels sprouts.

THE MEDITERRANEAN LIFESTYLE FOR ALL STAGES OF LIFE

In addition to what you're eating, how you live your life day to day has a profound effect upon your body and spirit. The Mediterranean lifestyle is important during all stages of life to optimize health, quality of life, and well-being.

DAILY PHYSICAL ACTIVITY

Routine physical activity can cut the risk of developing any major chronic disease *in half.* It has also been shown to improve cognitive performance in previously sedentary older adults, and is associated with overall psychological well-being. Kids should be physically active for at least 60 minutes every day, with at least three days of vigorous activity per week. Adults should strive for 30 minutes or more of moderate physical activity every day, getting in at least 150 minutes per week (or 75 minutes of vigorous exercise). During periods of prolonged sitting, get up at least once an hour and move around.

WEIGHT CONTROL

Being overweight adversely affects virtually every system in your body, so maintain a healthy weight. If you are overweight, losing even just a few pounds can be a profound benefit. Knowing your waist circumference is the best gauge for healthy weight, as it assesses the amount of abdominal fat you have, the most harmful kind. I have never had a treatment failure with patients who started the Mediterranean diet, be it for weight loss or maintenance.

COMMUNITY

La famiglia, sempre insieme—the family, always together. Among communities with the most centenarians across the globe, including in my Mediterranean town, we put our families first. Studies have shown that those with the most social connections of any kind live longer—be it ties to a spouse, relatives, friends, or through club membership, or volunteerism. It reduces stress and provides help of all kinds when you need it. Make an effort in this regard, and it will benefit you many times over.

CULINARY ACTIVITIES

Growing up, we were always in the kitchen, around the table, tasting and cooking. It was as fundamental as the Mediterranean Sea to our way of life. These activities provide social support and create a sense of unity. We were decidedly aware of food and appreciated it; it wasn't mindless snacking and gorging in front of the TV.

STRESS MANAGEMENT

These days we are under constant stress—hectic schedules, work pressure, traffic, pollution, and so on. Your body thus constantly senses it's under attack. The long-term activation of the stress-response system—and the subsequent overexposure to cortisol and other stress hormones—can disrupt almost all of your body's processes. Manage stress by engaging in relaxing activities and getting plenty of sleep.

SUNSHINE

Vitamin D, a vitamin our skin manufactures when it's exposed to the sun, is crucial for strong bones, healthy body function, and the prevention of chronic disease such as cancer (especially of the colon), cardiovascular diseases, and autoimmune disorders. Populations most at risk of vitamin D deficiency are those living in northern climates, those with dark complexions, children, and the elderly. The few dietary sources available include fatty fish and fortified milk and cereal. Get at least 10 to 15 minutes of sun exposure twice weekly (without sunscreen).

SUFFICIENT SLEEP

Sleep influences every organ, since most of the body's regenerative work happens while you are out for the night. Sleep deprivation is also linked to elevated levels of the stress hormone cortisol, which can lead to systemic inflammation and may underlie the development of many diseases as well as weight gain. Babies require up to seventeen hours of sleep a day; young children, ten to fourteen hours; grade-school-age children through adolescents, eight to eleven hours; and adults, seven to nine. Most adults age 65 and over still need seven to eight hours of shut-eye a night. As you age, you need about an hour less sleep a night (and don't sleep as well), but sleep is even more important.

WHAT NOT TO EAT

If you are eating a Mediterranean diet for snacks and meals, there will simply be less room for the things that aren't good for you. Don't weaken the benefits of the Mediterranean diet and sabotage your health by including too much of the following.

TRANS FATS

PROBLEM: Trans fats lead to the worst blood-lipid profile a fat can generate, raising bad LDL cholesterol and triglycerides while suppressing good HDL cholesterol. It's been linked to many conditions, such as diabetes, heart disease, and systemic inflammation. Manufacturers are authorized to list trans fats as "0" even if a product does contain trans fats, as long as it has less than 0.5 grams per serving. But this adds up if you eat the product regularly or consume a variety of items that contain it.

WATCH OUT FOR IT IN: Commercially produced foods (look for "partially hydrogenated oil" on the label), such as crackers, cake and frosting mixes, bottled salad dressing, frozen dinners, microwave popcorn, prepared cookie dough, pudding, beef sticks or jerky, ice cream, breakfast sandwiches, baked goods, nondairy creamers, deep-fried foods at restaurants, shortening, piecrust, margarine.

SATURATED FAT

PROBLEM: Too much saturated fat in the diet produces elevations in blood cholesterol levels, which translate into increases in the risk of cardiovascular and many other diseases. Some saturated fats have been shown to be neutral; however, none have been found to be health promoting.

WATCH OUT FOR IT IN: Red meat and other animal fat; dairy fat like butter, cheese, and cream; palm or palm kernel oil.

EXCESS OMEGA-6 POLYUNSATURATED FATS

PROBLEM: Omega-6 fats have generally been found to be heart healthy, especially when consumed as a replacement for saturated fat and when balanced with a high amount of omega-3 fats; however, excessive amounts are linked to many diseases.

WATCH OUT FOR IT IN: Poultry fat, corn oil, safflower oil, sesame oil, soybean oil, sunflower oil, and commercially made foods that use these oils.

HIGH-FAT DAIRY

PROBLEM: Whole-fat dairy supplies a higher calorie count and saturated fat and cholesterol content, together with no established nutritional advantage over low-fat dairy, so most dietary guidelines and scientific organizations recommend low-fat or nonfat dairy products.

WATCH OUT FOR IT IN: Cheese, ice cream, butter, whole milk.

PROCESSED MEAT

PROBLEM: Probably due to a high salt, nitrite, and nitrate content, processed meats are associated with significantly higher incidence of heart disease, diabetes, and pancreatic cancer in adults when compared with unprocessed red meat, and they have been shown to increase the incidence of leukemia in children and teenagers.

WATCH OUT FOR IT IN: Bacon, cured sausage, jerky, lunch meat, salami, pepperoni, hot dogs.

ALSO AVOID

Overcooked meat—It creates toxins.

Too much protein (especially animal-based)—It raises the risk of dying from cancer and all causes for those under age sixty-five.

Refined carbohydrates—Fiber and nutrients are processed out, leaving starch that's mostly empty calories and usually processed with more unhealthy ingredients.

Too much sugar—It's highly linked to many serious conditions such as heart disease, dementia, and inflammatory diseases, as well as excess weight.

Too much salt—It increases blood volume, causing high blood pressure and putting excess demands on the heart.

Pesticides—Many may be carcinogenic; children are most sensitive.

Dangerous food additives—Of the 10,000-plus chemical additives being used in the food supply today, only around 1,500 are FDA-approved; to keep up to date, check out the Center for Science in the Public Interest's website (www.cspinet.org).

Fast foods—They often have all of the above.

GOING MEDITERRANEAN AT ANY AGE AND BUDGET

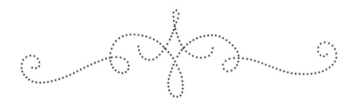

For most people, it's easy to start eating Mediterranean and adapting the diet to your lifestyle. The cuisine is so varied, there is something for everyone, and it's a cinch to get creative and prepare things to your taste. It helps that with Mediterranean cooking, instead of feeling like you're missing out while eating healthy, you'll feel sated and indulged.

Some may have a little trouble embracing every aspect, however, such as letting unhealthy habits go. In this section, we'll discuss common obstacles like how to reduce meat in your diet, how to find substitutions for unhealthful foods, how to follow the Mediterranean diet on a budget, how to save time when preparing food so you're not dependent upon commercially made foods, and how to cajole children into trying and liking Mediterranean cuisine (it's not as hard as you might think!). Changing habits is only challenging in the beginning—then they become your new go-to way of life.

SEVEN STEPS TO CHANGING YOUR HABITS AND FLAVOR PREFERENCES

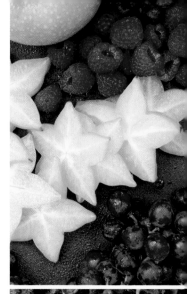

1. TAKE A WEEK AND TRACK WHAT YOU CONSUME EVERY DAY. Once you are aware of what you're eating, you may be surprised by the unhealthy foods and drinks you don't count in your mind.

2. ALLOW TIME TO CHANGE GRADUALLY. Forcing yourself to transform all at once likely won't last. Make one change at a time, adding healthy elements little by little. For example, to reduce meat, fold veggies into ground meat to lower the percentage of meat, use plant proteins and fiber-rich produce and whole grains to augment that full feeling, and use meat as an accent rather than the centerpiece of a meal. With high-fat dairy foods, progressively reduce the fat percentage. A taste for salt is readily reversible, just reduce salt slowly over time; avoiding processed foods will cut down your intake significantly. You might want to try salt substitutes like potassium chloride, as they don't have the undesirable health effects of sodium chloride (table salt), though people with kidney failure, heart failure, or diabetes, or those who take certain medications should not use salt substitutes without medical advice.

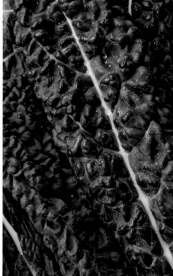

3. KEEP TRYING. Studies show that the more you eat something, the more you will like it. Have patience, and your preferences will change and cravings for unhealthy foods will fade away. Taste is instinct, but it's also habit.

4. EXPERIMENT. Taste fruits, vegetables, whole grains, nuts, seeds, and seafood you haven't tried before to expand the healthy choices you enjoy.

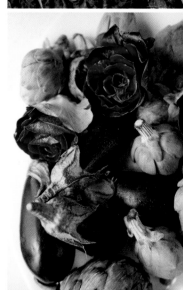

5. MAKE HEALTHY SUBSTITUTIONS IN YOUR FAVORITE RECIPES. Try using fish or skinless chicken—or, better yet, legumes or vegetables—in place of beef, use olive oil in place of butter, sauté instead of fry, use a sprinkle of cheese instead of slathering it on, have tomato-based sauces instead of cream-based, and so on.

6. INCREASE THE AMOUNT OF FRUIT YOU CONSUME. Add fruit to things you already eat, such as cereal, yogurt, or salads; eat it as a snack or dessert.

7. SEEK OUT IN-SEASON LOCALLY GROWN PRODUCE, OR GROW YOUR OWN. It will be much more flavorful and enjoyable.

HOW TO GET YOUR KIDS EATING THE MEDITERRANEAN DIET

JUST HAVE THEM TRY IT. It will be welcome news to parents that half the battle in converting children to the Mediterranean diet is to just get them to take a taste. Though there are some strongly flavored foods that are part of this cuisine, there are even more mild flavors that children will find appetizing. Some options bursting with nutrients that children usually find tasty: avocados, broccoli, brown rice, cheese, eggs, mild-flavored fish like salmon and cod, kidney beans, yogurt, pasta, a seed or nut butter, potatoes, poultry, squash, and sweet potatoes. Fruit is always a terrific way to get kids eating healthfully, as they are naturally drawn to its sweetness.

START SERVING NUTRITIOUS FOODS AS EARLY AS POSSIBLE. It's best if the Mediterranean diet actually begins in the womb. It appears that the flavors a mother eats wind up in the amniotic fluid and can be detected, thus commencing the development of taste preference. This foundation can then build upon itself, as foods babies become partial to show up in the food choices they make in later childhood, and as young children become increasingly resistant to change.

When I was growing up, there were not grocery store aisles devoted to countless jarred and packaged baby foods. Instead, we were given the foods the adults were eating, mashed up to a soft consistency. My wife essentially did the same thing for our children. She would put most everything we had on our table into the food processor as soon as they could start eating soft food. As a result, and true for me too, we developed a broad palate; my kids and I have liked vegetables ever since we were young, as well as fruits. The familiar evolved into a comfort food. For the Italian child, Mediterranean choices are comfort foods, and they crave them. Though as you'll see below, it's never too late to start.

BE PATIENT. It's natural for kids to be averse to unfamiliar foods. However, if they are introduced to new flavors slowly over time, they will frequently warm up to them. Research has shown that children often learn to like new foods after five to ten exposures, so gentle persistence can be key. If you keep giving them the old standbys, they're not going to branch out and explore new foods.

The best kind of learning happens in a positive atmosphere, often as a part of everyday life. Acknowledge good choices and good eating behavior: "I like that you chose that piece of fruit for your snack" or "I'm so proud that you're learning to make healthy food choices." (Note: Avoid praising them for how much they eat, as that could link approval to eating and overeating.) Nonfood rewards are fun to offer, such as stickers, marbles, longer story time, and so on. Start out easy: perhaps give a reward merely for tasting.

MAKE IT FUN. I like to slice and peel fruits for the kids and let them put the pieces on their plates in patterns. There are also cutting gadgets that turn veggies into zigzags, spirals, flowers, and other shapes. Children will be more inspired to adopt better habits if they're so distracted by the fun they're having, they don't even notice the food they're enjoying is healthy.

INVOLVE YOUR KIDS. Even at three years old, the more kids participate in the food process, the more conscious of good nutrition they'll be.

Kids get more interested in eating food that they've helped choose and make. Welcome them into the kitchen to help in whatever way they're able to for their age. Go to a farmers' market and choose all the parts of a dinner together, or start with one healthy item and decide together how you'll prepare it and form a meal around it. If they don't like something, ask them for ideas and flavors to add to make it taste better to them.

EDUCATE YOUR CHILDREN ABOUT NUTRITIOUS FOOD. Around two years of age, children can understand what's a treat and what's not. By age three or four, they can distinguish healthy from unhealthy food, and grasp what makes it so. By talking about healthy food and healthy choices beyond dinnertime, you show you care about them, and that helps your children care about them, too. One

Games to Try

Play longest/biggest/tiniest games: Who has the longest green bean? If yours is shorter, you have to eat it.

Play blind-taste guessing games: What is it? What flavors can you taste?

Hold crunch competitions: Who can crunch the loudest? Can you guess the crunch?

Have a color-finding mission in the produce aisles: Give each child a color or two and have them find something to bring home.

Do a rainbow challenge: Who can eat the most colors on their plate?

Play a "How does the food grow?" game: For example, *on vines* = grapes, tomatoes, kiwi, and melons; *underground* = carrots, potatoes, onions, beets, peanuts; *on trees* = olives, apples, pears, cherries, bananas, oranges, grapefruits, peaches, coconuts, lemons, mangoes, plums, avocados, pomegranates, cocoa beans; *on stalks* = corn, Brussels sprouts, pineapples; *as flowers* = artichokes; *straight up out of the ground* = asparagus, celery, leeks; *on bushes* = blueberries, raspberries, cranberries.

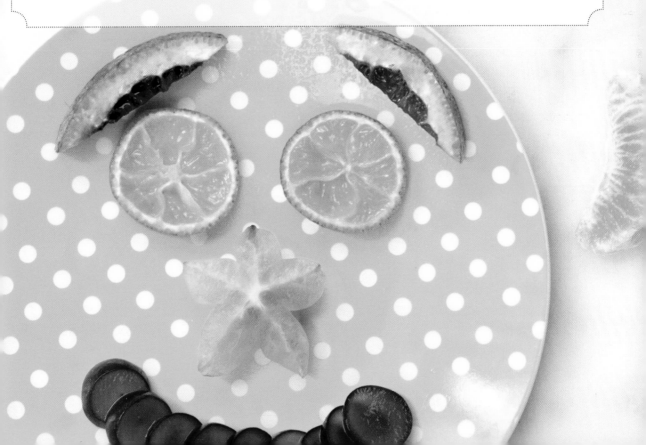

Advice for the Pickiest Eaters

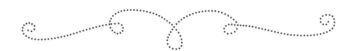

- **Add** grated or chopped vegetables to favorite foods. Try sprinkling grated carrots over cottage cheese, or spreading cream cheese on bread, and stirring diced zucchini into pasta or grated zucchini into pancakes.

- **Sauté** vegetables rather than serving them raw—they're usually sweeter that way.

- **Experiment** with different textures and tastes. Try different pasta shapes; present carrots grated, chopped, or boiled, or as raw baby carrots; serve cooked broccoli pureed as mash or soup if they don't like the florets.

- **Make** a smoothie together, letting kids pick the fruits and taste-test along the way to design one they like.

- **Give** them the power of choice, but only among certain options, such as which fruit or which vegetable.

- **Bake** recipes that contain veggies, such as pumpkin muffins or carrot bread.

- **Refrain** from telling them something is "healthy" while you're serving it. In the moment, most kids just want it to taste good.

- **Offer** the new food at the beginning of the meal when they're hungriest.

- **Surprise** them by turning things around. Breakfast can be for dinner, or dinner for breakfast. Picky eaters will eat more if that's what they're in the mood for, and the novelty of it makes it fun.

- **Make** a "try bite" chart with names or pictures of things they've tried, and they can put a smiley face, frown, or plain face (or whatever they choose) next to it to show how they felt about it.

- **Remember,** little ones have little tummies. Unless they're underweight, it's usually okay to respect their hunger cues.

good teaching arena is the supermarket. Talk to them about different foods and answer their questions. When they beg you to buy unhealthy foods or beverages, use it as an opportunity to teach them how to be wise shoppers. Perhaps allot them a little money to choose something healthy instead and talk through their suggestions.

KEEP HEALTHY FOODS STOCKED AND ON HAND. You are in charge of the foods that enter the house. Everyone eats what's available. Don't expect your kids or yourself to have willpower—most of us don't. If you're out of chips and they're hungry and apples are in a bowl on the kitchen counter, you have won the battle for a healthy snack. As for meals, stock up on nutritious staples so you can prepare healthy feasts in a flash (see "What to Have on Hand," page 74).

USE A LITTLE TOUGH LOVE. Sometimes it's appropriate to employ gentle coaxing, sometimes it's appropriate to negotiate, and sometimes it's time for a little tough love. I have patients tell me all the time that they can't get their child to eat this or that. The child says, "I don't want it," so parents say okay and acquiesce. "My kids won't eat anything but chicken fingers!" they'll say. Kids will push you and test their boundaries: they know you want them to be happy. It's hard to say no.

When my children push back and say, "Papa, I don't like this," I encourage each of them with what is most meaningful to him or her. For example, my boys want to grow up to be strong, so I tell them that. Sometimes they'll ask, "Papa, does this make you strong?"

"Yes, of course. This is what Papa eats. This is how Papa became strong."

My daughter, on the other hand, wants desperately to grow up to be tall like Mama, so that is the line of encouragement I offer to her. Do they want to be able to run faster? Play football? Avoid teasing at school? You have to know what they want and support them in that way.

My daughter went through a phase where all she wanted to eat was white pasta. We did not give in, though, and the phase passed.

When I was a teenager, I went through a phase like that myself. I decided I disliked minestrone soup. It was a dish my mother made frequently, full of wholesome ditalini pasta, an assortment of vegetables, and cannellini beans, and I developed an aversion to it. However, my mother didn't make anything different for me. If I was hungry, I had to eat it. Undoubtedly, because of her unrelenting approach I eventually developed a taste for it again, and today it's one of my favorite foods. You can't become a short-order cook for your children. If you do, you won't allow them the chance to develop a liking for a broad range of healthy foods.

DON'T RESTRICT TREATS ALTOGETHER. Research shows that not allowing children to eat certain foods only *increases* their desire for those foods. Help children learn that healthy foods like fruits and vegetables are "all-the-time foods" or "green-light foods" that they can eat anytime (if they're old enough, you can say they don't even have to ask), and that foods like candy, soda, cookies, and sugary cereals are "sometimes foods" or "red-light foods" that they have to ask for and can eat once in a while.

The advice to not restrict is even more true for teenagers. Strict rules about foods will likely backfire with them, and the fact is, you have less control because they are away from you more at this age. The importance of nurturing good habits at home is heightened, so if they eat the occasional fast-food meal out, it won't matter as much. Don't fret; they will likely come back around as they mature.

BE A GOOD ROLE MODEL. With kids, values are not so much learned as *absorbed*. If you want to improve your children's healthy habits, the best way is to model it as parents. "Do as I say, not as I do" rarely works.

Studies show the powerful effect of parental modeling of healthy behaviors on their children. Parents who are themselves willing to eat more fruits and vegetables will be more likely to have children who eat more fruits and vegetables. For example, children eat even fewer vegetables if the parent does not eat vegetables yet admonishes the children to do so. Eat healthfully, keep active, and show your excitement and enjoyment about your healthy lifestyle. This raises the likelihood that your child will want to live that way too.

TIPS FOR SAVING MONEY ON THE MEDITERRANEAN DIET

- Stock your pantry with inexpensive healthy staples (check labels of packaged products to ensure there are no undesirable additives):

sweet potatoes, peanut butter, oatmeal (steel-cut or rolled oats are best), brown rice, chickpeas, canned tuna, dried legumes, canned corn.

- Buy fruits and vegetables in season; they're cheaper then. If they're local, you're not getting charged for their transportation and storage costs, either.
- Freeze in-season fruits and vegetables for later, or buy frozen from the supermarket during the off season.
- Though not optimal, canned fruits and vegetables are still nutritious and cost less than fresh; just watch out for the liquids they come in, as they may contain sugar or salt. If so, it is best to rinse them off before use.
- Save the more expensive extra-virgin olive oil for cold dishes or for flavoring at the end of hot dishes, since you lose some of its nutritional benefit during cooking when the antioxidants start degrading. You can use refined olive oil or canola oil when cooking.
- When you eat good fat, protein, and fiber and drink plenty of water, you'll feel full longer and won't have to buy as much food and so many snacks.
- Canned tuna, salmon, and mackerel—on a sandwich, in a salad, or in a pasta dish—are inexpensive ways to put fish on your plate.
- What you won't be buying will save you money: cut back on or cut out sugary drinks, beef, potato chips, ice cream, doughnuts, sodas, your morning latte with three pumps of sugar syrup, and so on.

TIME-SAVING TIPS

In the US and many other places, the modern trend is for increasingly quick and solitary meals. Ready-made food is everywhere, with its healthfulness often sacrificed for convenience. The traditional Italian way—often still practiced to this day—is for school and work to be released at midday so everyone can go home for a long, freshly prepared family meal. I encourage you to prioritize taking time to cook and share meals with good company. You'll see that many of my recipes are

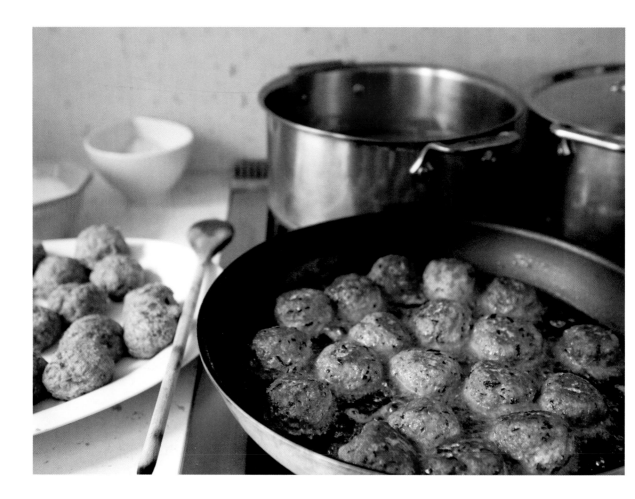

quick and easy already, and below you'll find tips to shave off preparation steps when you're tight on time.

TIME IS MONEY (WHAT TO GET AT THE GROCERY STORE)

- Buy high-quality ingredients—like fresh fish, extra-virgin olive oil, and authentic San Marzano tomatoes—and let their tremendous flavor do the work so you don't have to.
- Keep fresh fruits and vegetables washed and readily available.
- Buy frozen berries so you always have wholesome fruit on hand.
- Buy boxes of single-serving nut and/or seed packages for snacks on the run.

- Buy precooked rotisserie chicken (check the oils it has been cooked with).
- Buy precut frozen or canned vegetables.

BATCH COOKING (SIMPLIFY BY PLANNING AHEAD)

- Plan your weekly menu in advance so you can shop once (eating the most perishable items earlier in the week).
- There's no need for fancy recipes if the meal features fish or lean meat: extra-virgin olive oil and a little salt and pepper are all that are really required for an excellent result.
- The freezer is your friend: make large batches of recipes like soups, sauces, and breads; freeze them in meal-size portions and thaw them as needed.
- Roast a chicken or turkey, slice it, then vacuum-pack it after it's cooled and use it as needed throughout the week or freeze it for future use.
- Make a one-dish meal like an omelet using skim milk, an assortment of veggies, and low-fat cheese (for breakfast and beyond).

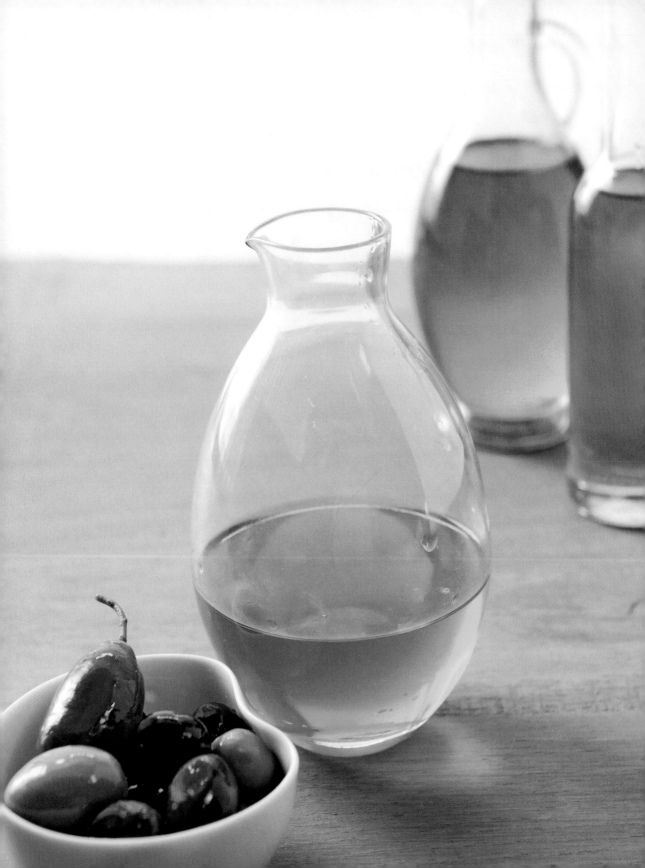

EAT SIMPLE

Mangiare Semplice

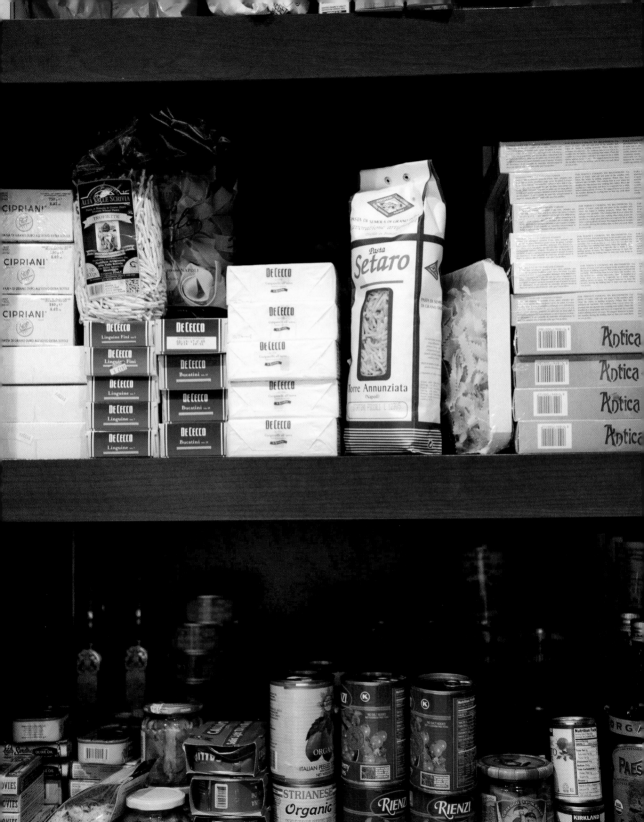

STOCKING YOUR KITCHEN
FOR THE WHOLE FAMILY

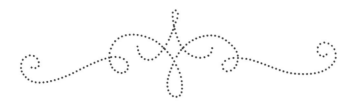

One of the most important tenets to remember about Mediter-
ranean cooking: good food begins with good ingredients. A
big part of what makes the Mediterranean diet so healthy—
and so delicious—is that meals are derived from fresh ingre-
dients, the fresher the better. Consequently, it can be tricky to
coordinate a series of meals without ending up with spoiled, wasted food. The
key is to have a cornucopia of items to choose from, both fresh and packaged for
a longer shelf life, and to do a little planning.

In Italy, people go to the market every day—they make it a priority, and it's
their routine. For many elsewhere, this prospect would not be convenient enough,
but I would recommend that you make an effort as much as you can. In addition
to the freshness factor, shopping for less food at a time keeps the fridge tidier and
prettier, creating inspiration when you open it, and making you less inclined to
forget about things that might otherwise go bad (which also saves you money). I
buy fresh bread daily, and buy fish daily or every other day. For fish in particular,

I choose the freshest available and build my meal from there, picking up any necessary fresh herbs or vegetables for sides. For example, just today I went to the fish store and was told that pompano had just come in, so I decided I would grill it and add lemon. Someone had given me black truffle paste, so I decided to use that, too, and bought fresh tagliatelle, and that was my meal. I enjoy trying new recipes, but day to day, my menu plan is inspired by what has just come from the ocean or garden.

I buy less perishable items at longer intervals. For example, I buy meat and chicken every three days, and vegetable, fruit, and other perishable staples every four to five days. Herbs I replace once a week. I always have carrots, celery, and Brussels sprouts available, and they can last for one to two weeks.

WHAT TO HAVE ON HAND

By taking a little time to stock your cupboards, pantry, and refrigerator well, you will always have the ingredients on hand to make a tasty meal in a snap. You can make any fish or chicken dish with a little olive oil, salt, pepper, and a dash of lemon—just add heat. If the fish happens to be freshly caught, you have an aromatic extra-virgin olive oil from southern Italy or Greece, and the salt and pepper are freshly ground, you'll have a five-star meal in your own dining room with as simple a preparation as they come. Experiment with my favorites listed below—and find your family's favorites.

STOCK YOUR REFRIGERATOR WITH . . .

SEAFOOD AND MEAT

Fresh seafood stored properly (see page 92 for details)	Lean meats
	Poultry

FRESH VEGETABLES

Artichokes	Brussels sprouts
Baby spinach	Carrots
Broccoli and broccoli rabe	Cauliflower

Celery

Cucumbers

Eggplant

Fennel

Kale

Mushrooms

Onions and potatoes (I keep
these in the refrigerator in the
summertime, as they last longer)

Radishes

Red, yellow, and green bell peppers

Salad greens

Scallions

Spinach

Swiss chard

Zucchini

FRESH FRUITS

Blueberries

Grapefruits

Grapes

Lemons

Limes

Oranges

Peaches (I keep these out if I want
them to ripen, and when they're
ready, I'll store them in the fridge)

Strawberries

DIPS AND SAUCES

Eggplant dip

Hummus

Olive Pâté (see page 190)

Tzatziki Sauce (see page 299)

FRESH HERBS
AND FLAVORINGS

Basil

Dill

Flat-leaf parsley

Ginger

Mint

Oregano

Rosemary

Sage

Thyme

Kitchen Herb Garden

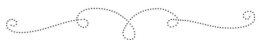

For exceptionally fresh herbs that cost next to nothing, grow them yourself. Beginning even in late fall,
you can grow them indoors during the winter in a
sunny window. Some are more suited for this than
others: try oregano, chives, mint, rosemary, and
thyme.

DAIRY

Eggs

Feta cheese

Grated Parmigiano or pecorino
  cheese

Low-fat milk

Low-fat yogurt

Ricotta cheese

STAPLES

Olives

Peanut butter and other nut butters
  (without trans fats)

Tomato juice and other juices (such as
  grapefruit and orange juices)

SWEETS

Jam (no sugar added)

STOCK YOUR FREEZER WITH . . .

Corn

Fava beans

Frozen fresh pasta like ravioli (it cooks
  quickly)

Frozen fruit for smoothies

Homemade chicken soup (frozen
  without pasta)

Homemade meatballs

Homemade minestrone soup (frozen
  without pasta, to be added when
  reheated)

Homemade pesto sauce

Peas

String beans

STOCK YOUR PANTRY WITH . . .

STAPLES

Bread crumbs (flavored and
  unflavored, traditional and panko)

Canned fish (anchovies, tuna,
  sardines, and mackerel packed in
  olive oil)

Couscous

Dried barley

Dried lentils and other legumes

Farina (Cream of Wheat)

Marsala wine

Oats (steel-cut or old-fashioned rolled)

Pasta of all shapes and sizes

Plenty of olive oil

Quinoa

Red and white wine

Rice (brown, long-grain, and wild)

Whole wheat and Italian breads (I like ciabatta and any type of Italian loaf with a nice crust that gives a crunch and isn't too doughy; store in a paper bag; best to get fresh daily)

Whole wheat flour

SPICES

Black peppercorns

Dried herbs (oregano, rosemary, sage, thyme, bay leaves)

Fennel seeds

Ground spices (cayenne, cinnamon, ginger, cumin, paprika)

Mediterranean sea salt

Red pepper flakes

SAUCES, DRESSINGS, AND FLAVORINGS

Balsamic reduction*

Capers

Clam juice

Dijon mustard

Horseradish

Ketchup (low sugar)

Soy sauce

Stock (vegetable and chicken stock)

Tabasco sauce

Vinegars (red and white wine, balsamic)

Worcestershire sauce

CANNED AND JARRED GOODS

Canned beans (such as cannellini, kidney, butter, chickpeas)

Canned whole plum tomatoes, diced tomatoes, and crushed tomatoes (with salt)

---

* For a richer flavor than balsamic vinegar in recipes, you can use balsamic reduction (also called balsamic glaze). You can find it in stores, or if you want to make it yourself, heat ¼ cup balsamic vinegar in a small pot over medium heat and reduce it by half (until it becomes creamy and has the consistency of maple syrup; add a little water if it gets too thick). It can be stored in an airtight container at room temperature.

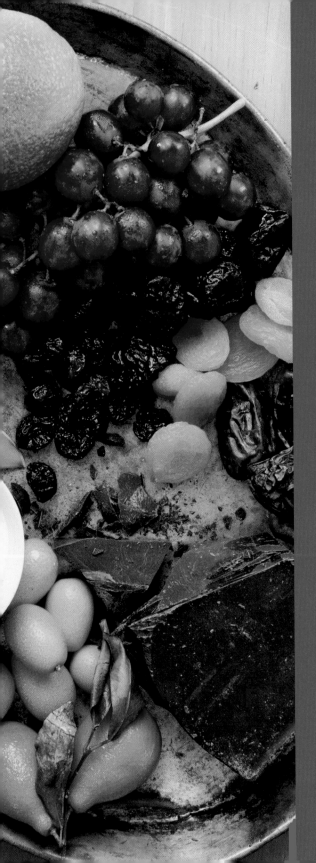

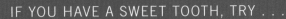
IF YOU HAVE A SWEET TOOTH, TRY . . .

- Fresh fruit (especially flavorful in-season varieties) and dried fruits
- Sliced pear topped with almond butter
- A couple of dark chocolate pieces with a stick of low-fat string cheese
- Banana "ice cream"—peel bananas, cut them into small pieces, freeze them for 1 to 2 hours on a plate, then use a blender to puree them to the consistency of ice cream
- Homemade fruit smoothie (e.g., a mixture of frozen fruit, yogurt if desired, perhaps a splash of juice for sweetness; see page 116 for recipes)
- Mixed nut crumble (page 286)
- Homemade frozen yogurt bar (combine your favorite low-fat yogurt with fresh fruit and freeze it)
- A banana or raspberries or strawberries (etc.) along with dark chocolate chips—these could be melted in the microwave for dipping
- Quick crumble—pop berries, pears, or apples into the oven (or even the microwave) with a touch of maple syrup and a dash of cinnamon on the top; when it's hot, sprinkle granola, oatmeal, or nuts over it as a crust

Approved Snacks

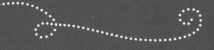

IF YOU'RE CRAVING SALTY, TRY . . .

- Nuts (try almonds, walnuts, pistachio) and seeds (try pumpkin, sunflower, squash seeds)
- Olives
- ½ ounce of Parmigiano cheese drizzled with 1 teaspoon of balsamic vinegar
- A piece of whole-wheat toast with extra-virgin olive oil drizzled on top
- Baked zucchini medallions with olive oil and grated Parmigiano on top
- Baked whole wheat pita chips or fresh veggies dipped in hummus, salsa, or Tzatziki Sauce (page 299)
- Chopped tomatoes sprinkled with fresh basil, lime juice, and a dash of salt and pepper
- 1 cup cherry tomatoes tossed with 1 ounce of crumbled feta, drizzled with olive oil
- Steamed edamame sprinkled with coarse salt
- Kale chips (take off the stems, lay the leaves flat on a baking tray, drizzle with olive oil, sprinkle with salt, and bake for 10 to 15 minutes at 350°F; add grated Parmigiano, red pepper flakes, or sweet paprika before baking for more flavor)
- Leftover homemade minestrone soup (pages 151–154)
- Homemade sweet potato chips, baked with olive oil and a pinch of sea salt

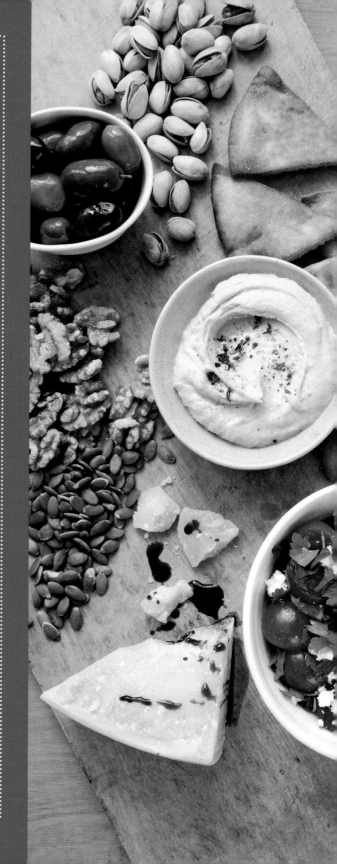

CANNED AND JARRED GOODS (continued)

Cornichon pickles (gherkins)

Sun-dried tomatoes (packed in oil)

Tomato paste

Tomato puree

Variety of other canned vegetables for
   backup (sans added ingredients
   like sugar, salt, and corn syrup)

DRIED FRUITS

Apricots

Cherries

Cranberries

Dates

Figs

Prunes

Raisins

NUTS AND SEEDS

Almonds

Cashews

Pine nuts (pignoli nuts)

Pistachios

Sunflower seeds

Walnuts

SWEETS

Brown sugar

Dark chocolate

Honey

White sugar

FRESH VEGETABLES

Avocados

Garlic

Onions (Spanish, Vidalia, red)

Potatoes (such as sweet, red, Yukon
   Gold, fingerling, Idaho)

Squash

Tomatoes

Turnips

FRESH FRUITS

Apples

Bananas

Pears

ESSENTIAL COOK'S TOOLS

While nothing in the world can quite compare to cooking with the finest and freshest of ingredients, these things can only be enhanced when you use the perfect tools for the job at hand. Like my mother always says, "The tools make the carpenter." When you have the right equipment and know how to use it, you can put your focus where it needs to be—on the food.

Chef's knife—Choose a 6-, 8-, or 10-inch knife (depending on the size of your hands, it should feel comfortable) for slicing meats and poultry and chopping vegetables, nuts, and herbs.

Cleaver

Dough scraper

Garlic press—My best friend in the kitchen! Choose one that works on unpeeled cloves and is dishwasher-safe.

Grater—I like the pyramid style with a handle.

Kitchen shears—Shears that easily disassemble make cleanup much easier.

Knife sharpener—Keeping knives sharp ensures that they're easy to use, quick, and safe. Every time I use a knife, I run it down a handheld sharpening rod beforehand. I also run all my knives through an electric knife sharpener once a week and get

them professionally sharpened every four months.

Ladle—Choose one with a bent handle at the top; this allows you to hook the ladle on the side of a pot so it won't fall in.

Lemon press

Locking tongs—Select a style with nonslip handles and scalloped tips for a firm grip.

Mandoline

Meat mallet

Metal spatulas

Microplane grater—For small tasks that require a fine grater, such as zesting lemons.

Oyster/clam knives

Paring knife—With its 3- to 4-inch blade, this knife is for smaller, precise tasks that require greater control (peeling, cutting, and carving fruit; mincing herbs or garlic; scoring meat).

Pasta grabber (or **pasta fork**)

Potato masher—A curved head will let you get into corners of bowls and pots.

Rubber spatula—Sturdy enough to maneuver heavy doughs but flexible enough to get into jar corners; silicone models are heat-resistant and can be used in pots on the stovetop.

Salt and pepper grinders—An easily adjustable grind setting will let you go from coarse to fine.

Serrated knife—Especially useful for slicing bread and tomatoes.

Skewers for grilling—If you use wooden skewers, you have to soak them in warm water for 10 to 30 minutes before threading or they'll burn up along with the food.

Slotted spoon—Stainless steel handles won't get too hot.

Spider—This is a wide, shallow wire-mesh basket with a long handle, used for removing hot food from a liquid or skimming foam off simmering broths.

Stainless steel pots and pans of various sizes—I prefer these because they're not reactive. For example, something acidic like tomato sauce reacts with uncoated aluminum, cast-iron, and copper pots, which can produce a metallic taste, darken light sauces, and shorten the life of the pan.

Vacuum sealer—For packing and storing meats and cheeses in the fridge and freezer.

Vegetable peeler

Whisk

Y-shaped vegetable peeler—This will give you a better grip than a traditional swivel model for hard-to-peel foods like mangoes and butternut squash.

EASY TIPS FOR BUYING, STORING, AND COOKING INGREDIENTS

Mediterranean cooking is home cooking. It's improvisational and very forgiving—use what you have on hand, substitute this for that, tailor it to your taste. This is not baking, where the measurements need to be ultra-precise; so if you're cutting down on salt, reduce the salt amount listed; if you're allergic to fish or don't have access to what I recommend, use another kind of fish or poultry instead.

In this section, I go into a little more detail about the ingredients I commonly use in the recipes that follow and provide tips for buying, storing, and cooking them. I've singled out the ones I use most and the ones people may be less familiar with, as well as the ones about which I have strong opinions or ideas about preparation that you may not have heard of before.

PRODUCE

BUYING

Sometimes it's hard to get excited about the bland-tasting fruit in today's supermarkets. This is often a result of the long journey to the store, as well as of commercial growers seeking to develop produce that lasts a long time. To that end, I recommend you try growing your own if possible. Local farmers' markets offering in-season produce are also a wonderful way to find the exhilarating taste of the perfect, sweet, ripe fruit.

Try to purchase in-season vegetables grown as nearby to you as possible. Let's spend some time focusing on key ingredients in these recipes.

THE ONION FAMILY

Experiment with different members of the onion family. They have potent anti-oxidants and contribute a range of flavors to recipes.

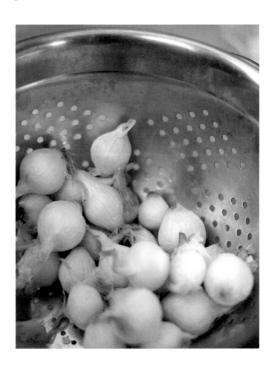

- VIDALIA ONIONS Sweet, good raw, and won't burn your tongue. I often use them on salads. I also like to sauté with them, because when you sauté, it brings out even more sweetness. I use a lot of Vidalia onions. Even though they're a little more expensive, they're worth it.
- SHALLOTS Interchangeable with onions, they're also on the sweet side and mild.
- SCALLIONS Milder than onions and often used as a garnish.
- LEEKS These look like large scallions and are sweeter than standard types of onions.

TOMATOES

When buying fresh tomatoes for cooking, I always get plum tomatoes, because they're meatier, firmer, and denser; they also have less water, fewer seeds, and lower acidity—all of these properties make them the superior choice for sauces. Smaller plum tomatoes are better. When they get very large, they're empty inside and not as flavorful.

The best region in the world for plum tomatoes (as well as cherry tomatoes) is the southern part of Italy. These prize tomatoes are grown in a region called San Marzano sul Sarno and are thus known as San Marzano tomatoes. I highly recommend that you use them when cooking with tomatoes.

The best canned tomatoes have the official Italian designation DOP—Denominazione d'Origine Protetta, or "Protected Designation of Origin"—printed on the label. In the case of tomatoes, the regulations that define them include:

In Sight, in Mind

Don't just keep fresh produce tucked away in a corner or fridge drawer. Instead, keep fruits on the top of an easily accessible kitchen table, along with dried fruits. That way, the family will grab them to snack on as they walk past, avoiding junk food.

- What strain of tomato they are
- Where in Italy they can be grown
- How they are to be grown
- The size, shape, and color when harvested
- That they are harvested by hand
- That they are peeled when packed

Note that just because a can says the tomatoes were packed in Italy doesn't mean they were grown there, even if it's a San Marzano strain of tomato. To ensure this you need to get DOP. The success of a tomato sauce such as marinara is all about the type of tomatoes you use (as well as blending the garlic into the sauce). Because canned tomatoes can vary greatly in taste, I stick to DOP certified. They may be double the price, but trust me, they're worth it. I prefer the La Valle brand.

When using tomatoes in salads, I am less particular and will use any kind—though I prefer them vine-ripened from a garden.

LEGUMES

Have a variety of both dried and canned beans on hand. Kidney beans and cannellini beans are staples. I also like butter beans; they are bigger and creamier than cannellini beans, and can be found at specialty stores. You used to have to go to specialty stores to find fava beans, but they're more readily available nowadays. I can often find them frozen at the supermarket.

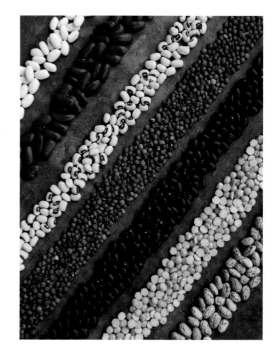

SQUASH

Try to buy squash with a 2- to 3-inch intact stem and without spots or bruising. It will last much longer. Squashes are a great staple to keep around because they're chock-full of nutrients and can last a long time without spoiling.

STORING

In Sicily we had fresh fruits and vegetables during the wintertime when not much was growing because we were able to store them effectively enough to last the three-month cold season. The rule of thumb was to leave the stems on. Removing a stem opens up a hole where air, moisture, and bacteria can pass through and cause deterioration. They also needed a cool, dry place and were suspended if the inside was more delicate. Onions we would store in a bushel in the attic, along with garlic, rolled up and hung. Cantaloupe could survive the winter as well if the stems were left on and they were suspended. Winter squash grew to seventy pounds and would be picked with the stem on. Grapes could last up to two months if left on the stems and hung. We didn't have a lot of space inside, so my mother would store and hang all of these foods in bedrooms and attics, wherever there was room—that gigantic winter squash was stored under the bed.

- TOMATOES Store these on the countertop, never in the refrigerator (the cold temperature destroys their texture and flavor).
- ARTICHOKES Store unwashed fresh artichokes in a plastic bag in the refrigerator for up to four days.
- EGGPLANTS Store them in the refrigerator; they become bitter with age, so use them in a day or two. Don't puncture or peel an eggplant, or it will perish quickly.

Washing Produce

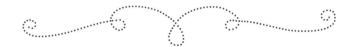

Pesticide residue tends to decline as the pesticide breaks down over time, and it diminishes as the produce is washed and processed prior to sale. By the time food reaches your grocery store, the residues are generally far below the legal limits. However, low levels may still remain on some foods, including organic foods. Even "prewashed" vegetables should be thoroughly washed. These tips will help you reduce pesticide residue (as well as dirt and bacteria) on the food you eat:

- Wash all produce (including what you plan to peel) under running water; flowing water is better than soaking or dunking.
- Dry produce with a clean cloth or paper towel.

- Scrub firm fruits and vegetables with a stiff brush.
- Discard the outer layer of leafy vegetables.
- If the produce was treated with wax, pesticide residues may be trapped underneath, in which case peeling is the most effective way to remove it (though you are then peeling off a very nutritious element, so try to buy wax-free produce).

For particularly dirty vegetables—like spinach, scallions, leeks, Swiss chard, and broccoli rabe—I first hold them under running water and try to loosen the dirt, then place them in a bowl of cold water to sit for a while until the dirt falls to the bottom; then I discard the water and repeat the soaking process two more times.

COOKING

It's important not to overcook vegetables, as they become mushy and unappealing, but undercooking can leave some vegetables raw and woody tasting. The absorption of nutrients into your body will vary with the style of preparation. Some vegetables are more nutritious raw; some more so cooked. Here's a quick guide to whether the raw or cooked version of some common vegetables offers the most health benefit:

VEGETABLE	RAW OR COOKED?
Asparagus	Cooked (steamed)
Beets	Raw
Broccoli	Cooked and raw
Carrots	Cooked and raw
Cauliflower	Cooked (but not boiled) and raw
Corn	Cooked (baked)
Eggplant	Cooked (baked)
Green beans	Cooked (baked)
Mushrooms	Cooked
Onions and garlic	Raw
Red peppers	Raw
Spinach	Cooked
Sweet potatoes	Cooked
Swiss chard	Cooked (baked)
Tomatoes	Cooked, best in oil
Zucchini	Cooked

Eat your vegetables from raw to cooked to benefit from all their various nutrients (except for deep frying, which adds too much fat, causes a loss of up to 50 percent of the nutrients available, and introduces toxins from the frying process). While cooking vegetables breaks down plant cell walls, making some nutrients and other phytochemicals more readily absorbable, most of the time, cooking them on high heat for short periods is best to preserve nutritional value. Microwaving, steaming, broiling, and stir-frying all fall into this category. Sautéing is a quick and easy way to cook vegetables with relatively little oil while preserving taste, texture, and color. Boiling vegetables, especially for long periods of time, will leach water-soluble vitamins out of them. If you do this, try to reuse the water for soups. Minerals are not as likely to be affected by cooking as vitamins.

When you are cooking with fresh **tomatoes**, recipes usually call for removing the seeds. This step is important because the seeds are bitter.

You have to be careful to not burn **garlic**, as it cooks very quickly. If it's whole, sliced, or crushed, you can put it in the pan along with the onion you are tenderizing for the same recipe (for two to three minutes), but if it's chopped or minced, it'll just burn, so you should put that in at the last minute. Alternatively, when onions are involved, you can sauté the onion for two to three minutes and then add the garlic. Another option is to cook the garlic in heated olive oil until it turns golden, then remove it before you add other ingredients. Its flavor stays with the oil.

As for **onions**, in my recipes, I usually suggest you add them to heated olive oil first and cook them until they are tender. Anything else you decide to sauté with the onion will turn a little bit sweet. And the more you sauté onions, the sweeter they become. If you don't do this, the onions take on a totally different flavor and are spicier. My motto: *Don't burn the onions*. You don't want to burn, brown, or caramelize them because it changes the flavor. I cook onions for only about 3 minutes. The onions in our recipes should be cooked enough to soften them and give the dish a sweet, creamy flavor. You can add a little water or white wine to the pan if they begin to burn.

Start cooking **potatoes** in cold water—it makes for a speedier cook time, ensures that they cook through, and imparts a better texture (no excess softening).

When prepping dried **beans** and **legumes**, either soak the beans overnight or rinse them and cook for a longer period of time to ensure they cook through. I do not add salt to the water while soaking.

PASTA

BUYING

In general, choosing a pasta type is a matter of taste and what goes well with the dish. By all means, experiment with different shapes and sizes. You'll develop your own feel for what you like. For example, in my opinion, if you have a plain tomato sauce, spaghetti is a great choice. Some people feel smooth tomato sauces work best with long, thin shapes like spaghetti, while chunky ones are better with a stubby shape with holes or cups to catch the sauce. I use penne rigati—the tubes with grooves on them—because the sauce gets in the ridges and makes the pasta more flavorful. Below are some suggestions for some pasta shapes with which you may be less familiar. Experiment and develop your own repertoire.

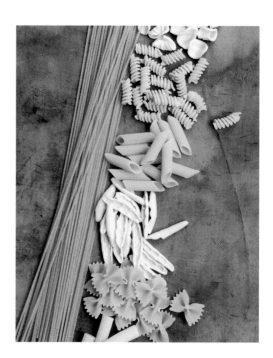

- DITALINI (small tube-shaped pasta)—Pair with small vegetables like peas or fava beans or in a soup, because it's easy to scoop into a spoon.
- FARFALLE (bow ties)—Pair with sauces when there are small pieces of meat to capture on it; children are entertained by the shape—it's like eating bow ties.
- LINGUINE (flattened spaghetti noodles)—Pair with seafood sauces.
- ORECHIETTE ("ears" in Italian; curved, circular pasta)—A kids' favorite, great for catching sauces.
- PACCHERI (large, ridged penne pasta from Puglia)—Pair with shrimp; great for dishes where you want the pasta to be more dominant.
- PERCIATELLI OR BUCATINI (spaghetti with a hole through the middle)—Pair with sauces that can flow through it, adding flavor.
- TAGLIATELLE (even flatter than linguine)—Pair with cream sauces.

STORING

Store dried pasta in a cool, dark place.

COOKING

SEVEN STEPS TO PERFECT PASTA

1. COOK PASTA IN A LOT OF WATER. When you drop pasta into a pot of boiling water, the starch granules on its surfaces instantly swell up and pop. The starch rushes out and, for a brief time, the pasta's surface is sticky with this exuded starch. Eventually, most of this surface starch dissolves into the water, and the pasta surface becomes slick again—this is what you want. To achieve it, boil pasta in a generous amount of water—4 to 5 quarts. It will come back to a boil faster when you add the pasta, and this helps to reduce sticking by quickly washing away the starch.

2. SALT THE WATER. I always add 1 to 2 tablespoons of salt to my pasta water (depending on how salty the other elements of the dish are). A generous amount of salt in the water seasons the pasta internally as it absorbs liquid and swells. The pasta dish may then require less salt overall.

3. STIR THE PASTA AS SOON AS YOU ADD IT TO THE BOILING WATER. To keep the pasta from sticking, you must stir it during the first minute or two of cooking. Otherwise, pieces of pasta that are touching may cook together.

4. DON'T PUT OIL IN THE WATER. There's no need to put oil in the cooking water to keep the pasta from sticking—no Italian does that. Just put the pasta into the vigorously boiling water. Stir it three times: as soon as you put it in, as soon as it boils again, and one more time during cooking. That's all you need to do. In fact, if you do add oil, you make the pasta too slippery for sauce to stick to it.

5. ALWAYS COOK AL DENTE. When you cook pasta al dente (firm to the bite), it tastes better, and it's better for you as well. If it's not as tender, it will require more chewing, which means you'll eat more slowly. That translates into better enzyme digestion and feeling fuller sooner. Overcooked pasta also sends blood sugar higher than pasta cooked al dente, which may contribute to subsequent cravings.

6. YOU MIGHT WANT TO RESERVE SOME PASTA WATER. I often reserve some of the pasta water after cooking my pasta if I'm preparing certain sauces for it. Pasta water contains the starch dissolved off the pasta, so you can use it to dilute whatever you're making and to achieve a nice, thick consistency.

However, I don't do this with tomato sauce because you need that to be nice and concentrated.

7. POUR THE PASTA INTO THE SAUCE, NOT THE SAUCE INTO THE PASTA. **Pasta** should be removed from its boiling water one minute before it is al dente, transferred immediately to the sauce that has been prepared for it, cooked for one minute longer in the sauce, then served right away. "You never, never leave the pasta sitting around in a colander," as one Italian cooking instructor has said. "In Italy, you could go to jail for that."

FISH AND OTHER SEAFOOD

BUYING

My hometown in Sicily, Castrofilippo, is located in the province of Agrigento, which is on the southern coast and was founded by the Greeks. I have very fond memories of going down to the seaside in the town of Agrigento, just fifteen minutes from my home, where the fishing boats came in with their daily hauls. You could have your fish prepared right there, not far from the boats. Octopus, sea urchins, mussels (we ate them raw), and so on—you can't get fresher than that unless you have your meal on the boat itself!

Alternatively, if you didn't get to Agrigento, Agrigento would come to you. Every morning, the fishmonger would drive around on his three-wheeled scooter yelling, "*Pisci! Pisci freeeee-schi!*" (or "Fish! Freeeeesh fish!"). You would meet him outside and buy it off the scooter. If the woman of the house was on the second floor when he came, she'd call down, say, "Give me two kilos of sardines," and send down a basket with money. She would then pull up the basket filled with her fresh sardines.

I know from experience that the best seafood is the freshest seafood. I get loads of compliments on the fish dishes I cook, and the simple secret is that I buy great fish. My purchase is always based on what's freshest at the fish counter. I can't go down to the Mediterranean Sea and bring home the catch of the day, but I get the closest to it that I can.

Many of the fish in supermarkets are farm-raised. They're all the same size and have a bland homogeneity to them, so I prefer wild fish. I can go to my fish counter and bring home wild branzino caught off the coast of Greece, and with the simplest of preparations, we eat a meal that tastes out of this world—it's the texture and flavor of the seafood that make the meal extraordinary.

Even at a general, landlocked supermarket, the fish attendants can tell you what they just got in. Get to know them at your local store; they are your best resource for procuring the freshest seafood possible.

Below I'll advise you on how to work with various types of seafood, some of which may be unfamiliar to you. I'll also share my best tips for cooking with seafood.

GENERAL FISH-BUYING TIPS

REGARDING THE STORE: It should have high-volume sales so you know turnover is high. It should smell like the sea (not fishy or sour), and the seafood should be stored on ice or well refrigerated.

REGARDING THE FISH: The flesh should be firm, not mushy (ask the fishmonger to press the flesh to confirm the texture); it should be moist and shiny, not dull; the eyes should be clear; and it should have a smell of the sea. Ask the fishmonger to cut it for you—it's easier for you, and it's better to not buy the packages of precut fish.

REGARDING LIVE SEAFOOD: When transporting anything living—such as mussels, clams, oysters, or lobsters—you don't want them put in a sealed plastic bag, because they'll die. You have to put them in a paper bag. A nice, wet cloth on top of the seafood would be helpful as well. You can place the paper bag in an unsealed plastic bag to manage leaks, or seal the plastic but poke holes in it.

REGARDING CANNED SEAFOOD: When buying canned seafood, it should always be packed in oil, otherwise it tastes like cardboard. I prefer Calipo tuna from Sicily. Please note that Italian canned seafood regularly comes in 6-ounce containers. For the purposes of my recipes, you can substitute American canned seafood that comes in 5-ounce containers.

ANCHOVIES

I use anchovies a lot when I cook, both for their tremendous flavor-enhancing quality and because they're so good for you with their concentration of healthy fat. It doesn't matter if they're canned or jarred. Sicilians use the ones packed in salt, but they're tedious to prepare because you have to then take off the salt and scales and fillet them. I prefer the ones packed in oil.

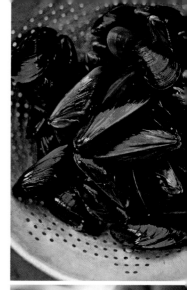

MUSSELS

Mussels should feel nice and heavy; if they feel light, it means they're not very good. Don't buy any that are open, because they are probably already dead. (If you do end up with open mussels, press them together to see if they'll stay closed. If not, they're dead—don't cook them.) Scrub and clean them before you cook with them by taking a handful and rubbing them together in your hands under cold running water.

SQUID

Squid are also known as calamari. Don't ever buy them frozen—they don't taste anywhere near fresh. They should also be firm, just like regular fish, so don't buy them if they're mushy.

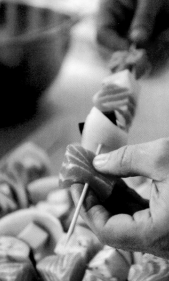

BRANZINO

Sea bass (sometimes called European sea bass) is what we refer to as branzino (plural, *branzini*). Along the East Coast in the US, it's striped sea bass, or black sea bass. It has a slightly sweet, mild flavor with a velvety texture.

SCALLOPS

"Wet" scallops are not as high quality as "dry" scallops. Wet scallops are soaked in salt water so they preserve better, but they have absorbed the water they soaked in, so essentially 20 percent of their weight is water, and you're paying for it. They will also

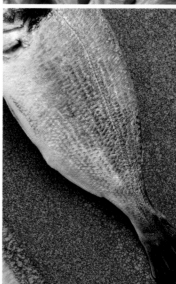

not caramelize as well in the pan. Few vendors carry the dry ones, and they're more expensive, but to me, they are worth the effort and expense.

SHRIMP

If you're buying shrimp to grill or eat plain, get the bigger ones (e.g., fifteen to twenty per pound); to put in pasta or another dish, get smaller ones.

TUNA

Tuna should be a deep red with a firm texture. The smaller the tuna, the better, because that means it's been in the ocean for less time and its body will have accumulated less mercury. This is true for any big ocean fish, such as swordfish.

SALMON

Farmed salmon has a higher fat content and is flakier, while wild-caught salmon tends to have a meatier texture with a finer grain. I always buy the salmon that is the freshest, regardless of whether it is farmed or wild.

SWORDFISH

The smaller the swordfish, the better, because that means it's been in the ocean for less time and will have less mercury.

STORING

When you store any kind of seafood, you want it to be maximally chilled without freezing. Fish spoils fast, partly because of its unsaturated fat—it's more prone to oxidation (unlike the saturated fat in other meats). Fish also live in very cold water, unlike warm-blooded animals, so the bacteria and enzymes in their bodies more easily break down in warmer temperatures. Store fish (fillet or whole) by washing it, drying it thoroughly, fully wrapping it in paper towels, then fully wrapping it, nice and tight, in plastic. If stored in this way, fish can stay in the refrigerator for about 48 hours without

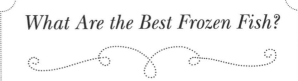

What Are the Best Frozen Fish?

None! Always buy fresh if you can. The only thing I buy frozen is shrimp.

starting to decompose and taking on a fishy smell. Keeping it on ice will preserve it even better; you can place the sealed bag on top of ice in a covered pan in the refrigerator (just make sure no water gets in the bag). Keep it in the coldest part of the fridge, usually the back.

If you're working with live seafood such as clams, mussels, oysters, lobsters, or other crustaceans, do not seal them in plastic, as you want them to stay alive until you're ready to prepare them. I store mussels, clams, or lobsters on a bed of ice and then cover them with a wet paper towel or wet cloth. Instead of ice, you can also just wet the cloth every day, getting it nice and wet so it doesn't dry out. The secret to storing live seafood is always keeping them moist. They will keep one to two days this way; clams will keep for three to five days. When the mussels and clams start opening, you know they're starting to die.

Don't clean mussels until right before you're ready to cook them; once their beards are removed (the strands sticking out where the halves attach), they die. Clams, however, you can clean beforehand.

COOKING

Always begin with a dry fish—pat it with a paper towel if it's damp. Timing is most important when it comes to cooking seafood. Perfectly cooked fish is moist and maintains a delicate flavor. Overcooked fish, on the other hand, is dry and unpalatable, so take care. Since fish are a bit fragile, a nonstick pan will make it easier, though a stainless steel or cast-iron skillet will render it crispier and more golden, so it's your choice. If the fish is less than ½ inch thick, it generally doesn't need to be flipped. It is done cooking when the flesh begins to turn from translucent to opaque or white and feels firm but still moist—it should be just ready to flake (cooking fish until it flakes easily risks turning it tough and dry). Removing fish from the heat source before it becomes opaque all the way through ensures that it will retain its moisture and remain tender.

When grilling fish, place the fish—dried, oiled, and salted—on a well-oiled hot grill. Do not touch the fish; be patient, because if you start to move it around too soon (before the skin crusts), it will stick to the grill. When grilling or baking a whole fish, you can tell when the fish is cooked by looking at the inner opening made to clean out the abdomen. When it dries, the fish is cooked. When broiling, I cook most fish skin side up to keep it moist, but salmon broils best meat side up. (And don't remove the gray meat near the skin—it's rich in omega-3 fat.)

Here are a few steps to aid you in preparing the different types of fish we'll be using:

- SCALLOPS   You want to keep scallops very dry before sautéing, and be sure not to overcook them.
- MUSSELS   Use your widest pot or kettle when preparing mussels, as this will allow the cooking liquid and steam to easily reach them. The trick to cooking mussels is not to cook them on a high flame. You have to cook them on a low to medium flame, stirring regularly; otherwise, they will open too quickly. You want them to be nice and plump. Once you put them into the pot, it should take 5 to 6 minutes for them to start opening, which is the sign that they're done. At this point, stir them, because the pressure of the mussels on top will keep those on the bottom closed. After this, they'll need another minute or two. Discard any that haven't opened after 6 to 7 minutes. Be careful not to overcook them, as they turn tough and tasteless.
- MACKEREL   This delicious fish cooks very quickly, in only 3 to 5 minutes. You don't want to overcook it, because that takes all the oil out.
- SQUID   When cooking squid, bear in mind that they are finicky and you need to pay particular attention so they don't get tough. If you fry them, they have to be nice and dry before you cook them; otherwise, they'll splash all over the place. You don't want to use very big squid for frying, as they're tougher. They should be dry before you flour them and the oil should be very hot, 375°F. Do not overcrowd the pan, as it will cool the oil. Fry for 2 to 3 minutes. Remove from the oil and place them on a paper towel, salting them as soon as they come out of the oil. Serve hot.

  To boil them, you can plunge them into boiling water and cook them for 2 to 3 minutes once the water returns to a boil—but if you don't take them out of the pot after that, you'll have to cook them for 20 to

30 minutes on a slow simmer to regain their tenderness. If the water comes to a rigorous boil during this longer cooking time, the squid will get tough and stay that way. Though they are finicky to prepare, squid are a favorite in Mediterranean cuisine. They can be presented in so many ways: with pastas, salads, and vegetables; in a sauce; or combined with other sautéed, stewed, or baked fish. When squid are served in a loose sauce, it is great for dunking bread.

To grill squid whole, make sure they're dry first, then put a couple of slits on the tubes to score them; place them on a well-oiled, very hot grill, and put a weight on them, like the bottom of a clean frying pan or a brick covered in aluminum foil. Grilling squid is quick, approximately one minute on each side. Salt the squid after it is cooked and it comes off the grill.

POULTRY AND MEAT

BUYING

Grass-fed beef is better for you, as it has more of the seemingly neutral stearic fatty acid, as well as more omega-3 fat, less omega-6 fat, and more vitamins, minerals, and antioxidants passed on from the grasses. Corn-fed beef is fattier, and though fat marbling adds to taste and tenderness, it has more of the harmful saturated palmitic and myristic fatty acids.

Avoid beef from dairy cattle, if possible—about 20 percent of American beef comes from this source. These cows have been injected their whole lives with drugs like growth hormones and antibiotics to help them produce copious amounts of disease-free milk. Unfortunately, there are no beef source labels at the supermarket. (However, beef labeled "Certified Angus Beef" is reliably from cattle raised specifically for their meat.) Even beef cows (except those labeled "organic") receive an implant in their ear that delivers hormones like estrogen to fatten them up.

The **beef** cuts I cook with most are sirloin and prime steaks. Loins and rounds are the leanest. When cooking with **veal**, choose chops and cutlets, and shoulder or neck for stew. Because veal can be lean, be careful not to overcook it. Veal cutlets only take one minute to cook on both sides. When cooking with **lamb**, choose rib chops and the leg. Different cuts of lamb take the same cooking time, especially if you are grilling. Stew meats, because they are cooking in a liquid, can be cooked for longer periods of time.

I prefer **natural, free-range chicken**, because it's tastier than other chicken. No need in my opinion to spend extra money on organic. On my farm, we let the chickens out in our fruit orchard, and they eat the fruit that drops from the trees, along with whatever bugs are on the grassy ground. All table scraps are given to the chickens. For some reason, they love any kind of pasta. Their meat is very juicy and flavorful.

STORING

Put fresh meat in the back of the refrigerator, where it's coldest, as soon as possible after purchase, as it will begin to bleed at warmer temperatures and the meat will become dry and tasteless. Go by the package directions for storage time. When I buy meat from the butcher, I don't keep it in the refrigerator for longer than two days.

Poultry and meat can be frozen, as the flavor does not change much, so I usually keep frozen chickens and steaks on reserve in my freezer. I store mine vacuum sealed, and they keep for up to three months. If you do not have a vacuum sealer, to prevent freezer burn, wrap individual steaks or chicken pieces tightly in plastic wrap and put them in a resealable plastic bag. You can freeze whole chicken in its original packaging.

COOKING

As with vegetables, sautéing chicken is a quick way to cook with relatively little oil. If you heat the pan, then add the oil and wait until it's hot; the hot oil causes the internal moisture in the food to boil and then escape as steam. The outward rush of steam prevents the surrounding oil from permeating the food and making it greasy.

When you grill meat, make sure the grill is lightly oiled and hot, and that the meat is dry before you put it on the grate. I can tell when steak is cooked by touching it to check the firmness: it is medium cooked when it has about the same firmness as the skin and muscle between my thumb and index finger. Try this tip, and after a while, you'll get used to the feel; it will take away the stress of guessing.

When cooking steak, I salt it after cooking to prevent the juices from being drawn out. However, I salt chicken beforehand. I usually cook it with the skin on to help maintain its moistness, then take the skin off before eating. Take care not to overcook chicken. When roasting, to give the chicken a nice golden color, I turn the oven to broil for the last three to five minutes. Let meat rest for five to seven minutes after removing it from the heat, as this allows the water pushed out during cooking to be reabsorbed, adding juiciness.

CHEESE

BUYING

In southern Italy, many people had their own goats and sheep and used the milk to make a variety of cheeses. We all made our own, mostly from sheep—this is called pecorino cheese—and we'd put pepper-corns in it. Ricotta is the first condensation before you make cheese; you skim it off the top, and it's very creamy.

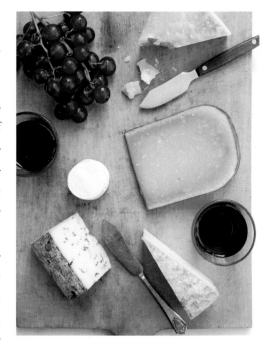

I love cheese. I add cheese to everything. However, as you'll notice in these pages, I don't have cooking advice for cheese. I don't pile it on—I use it as an accent and flavoring, adding it to dishes in slices, as crumbles, or grated. Grating is especially satisfying. This makes it look like more than it actually is. Parmigiano (the king of cheese in Italy), pecorino, Parmigiano-Reggiano, and Grana Padano are all favorites. If you get aged Parmigiano, it's more flavorful. Parmigiano-Reggiano and Grana Padano cheeses are hard, granular cheeses, while pecorino is soft. I get my cheese fresh from a cheese counter. I prefer full-fat ricotta. The low-fat version doesn't have the creamy texture that I like, and I don't use very much ricotta. However, if you're watching your fat consumption, low-fat ricotta is an alternative.

STORING

It is worth it to invest in a vacuum sealer to preserve cheese longer and prevent mold growth. If you do not have a sealer, wrap the cheese tightly in plastic and keep it refrigerated. Buy large chunks of the hard cheeses. You can grate them and store them in the refrigerator in a tightly sealed plastic tub or wrapped well in plastic. They will keep for two to three weeks. Ricotta lasts about five days in the fridge.

OLIVE OIL

BUYING

Since it's the combination of the oil and the antioxidants that gives olive oil its all-star nutritional status, one must choose the "extra-virgin first-cold-pressed" variety in order to take full advantage of its health benefits. "Extra-virgin" means the oil is extracted by crushing, not by using chemicals (as most other oils are), and must meet taste standards. "First-pressed" means that the fruit of the olive was crushed only one time to obtain the oil, and "cold" refers to the temperature range of the fruit at the time it's crushed (higher temperatures allow more oil to be extracted, but the quality and nutritional value suffer). With modern technology, the olives are not literally *pressed*—they used to be pressed between porous mats—but the terminology still refers to the first crushing.

My favorite olive oils are from Sicily because they're more flavorful and fragrant, like Letizia extra-virgin olive oil. Another one I love is Lu Trappitu, also from Sicily. Both are certified DOP. I prefer strongly flavored olive oil, but you may differ—experiment.

What to Look for
When Choosing Olive Oil

- Choose "first-cold-pressed" extra-virgin olive oil.
- Check the bottle for its harvest or milling date and buy the freshest possible. A dark glass bottle helps slow the oil's rate of oxidation.
- Note that "light" or "extra-light" doesn't refer to calories but to extra processing and refining. Extra-light oil has essentially no color or flavor (or healthy phenols).
- "Packed in/imported from . . ." designates where the olives were bottled or shipped from, not necessarily where they were grown. If the imported-from country is not the country of origin, the true "birthplace" is supposed to be listed somewhere on the bottle.
- Small producers (without the middlemen, who buy from a wide variety of producers to sell to corporate buyers) may be more likely to be selling authentic extra-virgin olive oil.
- The California Olive Oil Council gives a seal if an olive oil passes their test of being pure extra-virgin olive oil rather than a blend of cheaper oils.

STORING

Olives used to be harvested and pressed toward the fall in southern Italy. The oil would keep for a year—because of its low oxidation rate, it also lasts longer than many oils—though it is much more fragrant and contains more antioxidants if freshly pressed. Open olive oil within a year and a half of the production date on the bottle, and use it up within a few months after opening to prevent as much oxidation as possible. Store it in a cool, dark place; never keep it near the stove.

COOKING

When you cook with olive oil, most times it's best to first heat the pan, then add the olive oil, and add the first ingredient to the pan after the olive oil is hot. You can tell when it's ready because it shimmers—you'll see little waves (you don't want to see bubbles). Don't wait until the oil smokes; you don't want it to burn, as it loses its health benefits and flavor.

Cooking at high heat for long periods of time will degrade olive oil, and you'll lose its health benefits. Heat contributes to the oxidation of any fat. The same qualities that give olive oil protective effects in terms of LDL oxidation, however, also protect it in cooking, so it has more heat resistance than many other vegetable oils. This also means that extra-virgin olive oil, with its antioxidants intact, will stand up better during cooking than refined olive oils.

To counter the reduced health benefits caused by cooking, don't use old olive oil that has already partially oxidized, periodically replenish the oil during the cooking process, and add the last bit of oil close to the end of the cooking time. I always drizzle fresh olive oil on top of cooked entrees and vegetables. My mother taught me this—she said it adds flavor, since cooked and fresh olive oils taste different.

A concern regarding cooking with oils is their potential to create harmful substances when frying. The danger occurs mainly when a food is fried in a vegetable oil, and toxins are released into the air in the smoke. For this reason, I recommend that you don't deep-fry (it's not healthy anyway) or cook above the smoke point (which is when a bluish smoke can be seen). Be sure your stove and kitchen are well ventilated.

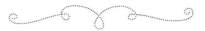

Take a Walk in the Real Olive Garden

In addition to getting lots of olive oil in your diet, take advantage of the wholesomeness of olives in their natural state as well. I encourage you to experiment with different kinds. Some people like different colors, different brines, different seasonings—it's all a matter of taste. Give this easy recipe a try. It's delicious.

SAUTÉED OLIVES

Serves 4

3 tablespoons olive oil

4 cloves garlic, crushed

2 cups large unpitted black olives (Kalamata or black oil-cured olives)

¼ cup red wine vinegar

1 teaspoon dried oregano

To a hot pan add the oil and garlic and sauté for 1 minute, then add the olives and vinegar. Cook over medium to high heat until the liquid has been reduced by half, then add the oregano. Serve hot with good Italian bread, your favorite cheese, and a glass of wine.

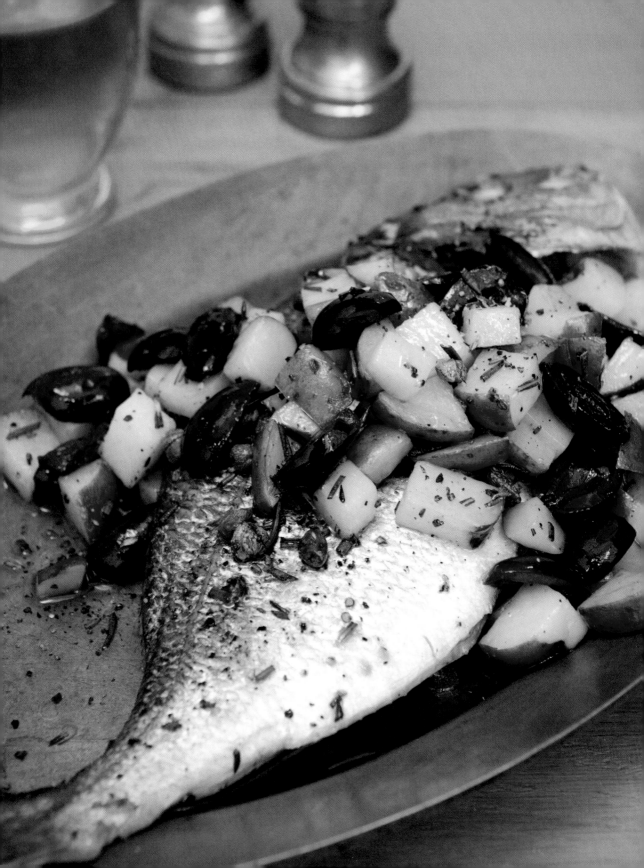

EAT WELL

Mangiare Bene

Now that you've come to understand the marvelous healthful-ness of the various components of the Mediterranean diet, I'll help you to put it all together and bring it into your life. With the recipes I've included here, you'll be able to make delicious, nutrient-packed dishes and meals that can be whipped up in surprisingly little time, proof that food that's good for you can also be beautiful, great tasting, and a joy to prepare, serve, share, and eat.

My path to the kitchen of course began in Italy, where they more or less put a colander in a newborn's hand instead of a rattle. I grew up in a family where daily life revolved around mealtimes and their preparation, as it did for most families in my community. My town was poor monetarily, but rich with fertile land to farm and copious delicacies from the sea a stone's throw away. Nothing was taken for granted. In devoting attention to our food, we were able to create sumptuous feasts with very modest resources.

My love of cooking was passed on to me from my mother, as well as from the culture at large, and absorbed, becoming a part of me. So much so that when I later moved to Manhattan, I bonded with many in the restaurant-chef community, where my zeal for food was shared. When I appreciate a meal, I make it a point to meet the chef, and so my circle of friends came to include those people who are as impassioned about food and its preparation as I am. Accordingly, you'll see that some of these recipes have been passed on or inspired by recipes from my favorite restaurants and dear friends.

I've also included icons with the recipes as a guide for particular age groups:

B = great for babies
K = kid-friendly
S = maximizes nutritional needs for seniors (age sixty and above)

Though the Mediterranean diet can be enjoyed by the entire family, the periods of infancy, childhood, and the mature years are times when people have specific textural and/or nutritional concerns. These highlighted recipes are brimming with ingredients that help fulfill those various needs. Bear in mind that if you eat a wide variety of the "Fabulous 14," you can't go wrong at any age.

Breakfast and Lunch

B babies
K kids
S seniors

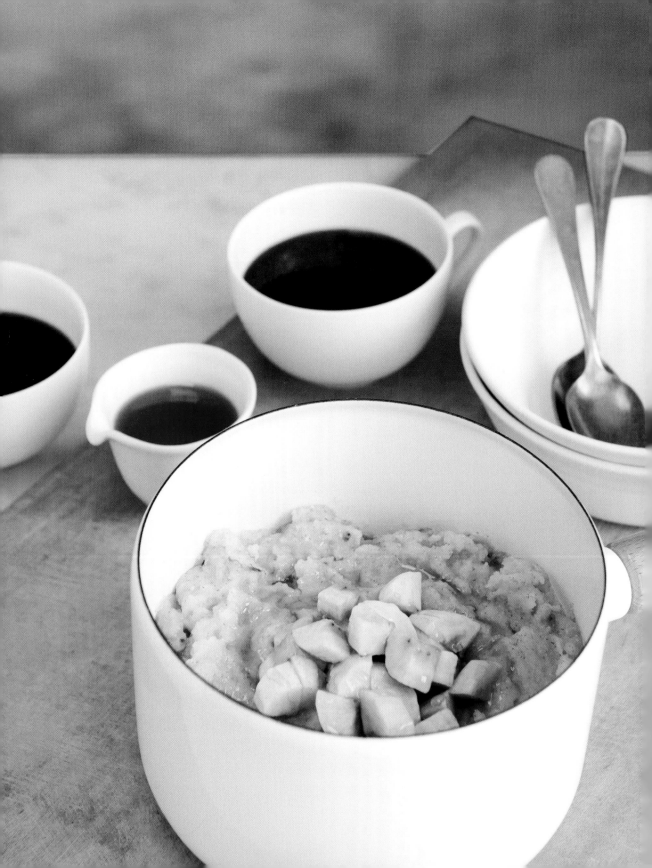

Farina with Fruit

B babies **K** kids

Farina is a cereal usually made from semolina and served warm; it is also known as Cream of Wheat. Kids can have fun helping make this and can add fruits to their taste.

SERVES 2

½ cup milk, plus more if desired
Pinch of sugar
Pinch of salt, optional
⅓ cup farina
1 banana, mashed
½ tablespoon honey (for ages
   1 and up) or maple syrup

½ cup fruit (ripened raspberries,
   blueberries, fresh or canned
   chopped peaches), optional
½ teaspoon cinnamon, optional,
   (see Note)

1. Combine ½ cup water with the milk, sugar, and salt (if using) in a small pot and bring the mixture to a boil over medium heat.

2. Add the farina while stirring and bring to a boil again, then lower the heat to a simmer. Cook for 2 to 3 minutes (you may add more milk to achieve your desired consistency), then remove the pan from the heat.

3. Mix the banana into the farina, along with the honey or maple syrup, and serve it topped with your choice of fruit and cinnamon, if desired.

NOTE: You get nutritional bang for your buck with cinnamon. It's loaded with antioxidants, has antimicrobial properties, may bestow neurological benefits and slow stomach emptying, and by mimicking sweetness, allows you to cut back on sugar.

BREAKFAST AND LUNCH   109

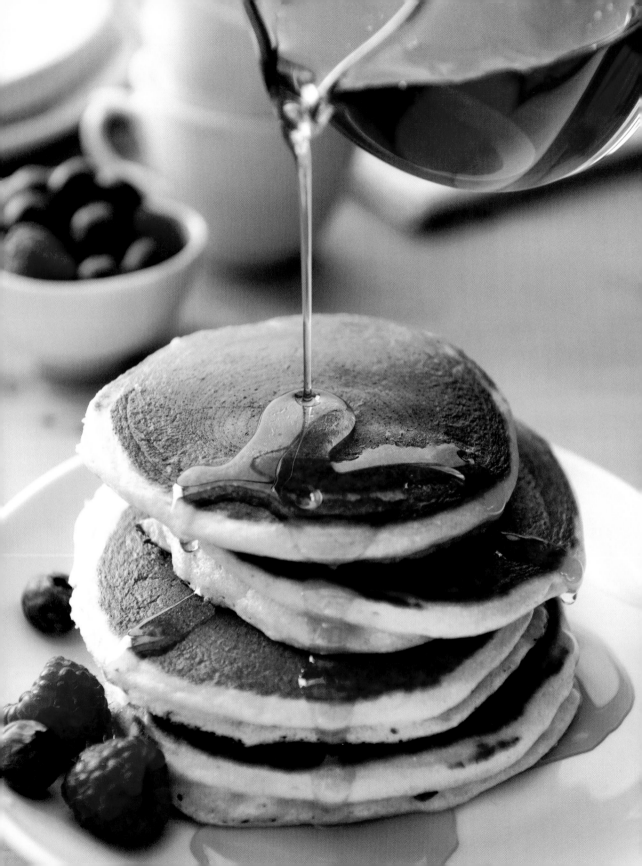

Ricotta Pancakes

This recipe will elevate your morning pancakes to another level.

SERVES 4

1⅓ cups all-purpose flour
1 teaspoon baking powder
¼ teaspoon baking soda
¼ teaspoon salt
1½ tablespoons sugar
½ cup ricotta cheese (I prefer
    whole-fat)

½ cup whole milk
1 tablespoon canola oil
2 eggs
Maple syrup, for topping
Berries, for garnish, optional

1. In a mixing bowl, combine the flour, baking powder, baking soda, salt, and sugar.

2. In a separate bowl, stir together the ricotta, milk, oil, and egg; mix well.

3. Combine the ricotta mixture with the dry mixture. Stir enough to remove all the clumps of flour, but do not overmix. Let the batter sit for up to 10 minutes.

4. Place a nonstick pan over medium heat. When the pan is hot, pour 1 to 2 tablespoons of batter per pancake (kids like their pancakes small) into the pan, spacing the pancakes far enough apart that they do not touch. Cook them for up to 1 minute per side, until golden brown.

5. Transfer the pancakes to a warmed plate and drizzle them with maple syrup. If desired, garnish with berries.

Scrambled Eggs with Olive Oil and Cheese

Ⓚ kids   Ⓢ seniors

If you have never made scrambled eggs with olive oil, you're in for a treat! Adding any kind of fat to scrambled eggs makes them more tender. Swap out that butter or margarine for heart-healthy olive oil, and you may be surprised how much you and your kids enjoy the flavor and texture.

SERVES 4

8 eggs
¼ cup whole milk
½ teaspoon salt
2 tablespoons extra-virgin
  olive oil

½ cup grated Fontina cheese, or
  any soft cheese

1. Add the eggs, milk, and salt to a large bowl and beat with a fork or whisk.
2. Place a nonstick pan over medium-high heat and add the oil and beaten egg mixture.
3. Sprinkle the top evenly with the cheese and mix it into the eggs with a rubber spatula.
4. Continue to stir gently, cooking for 1 to 2 minutes, until you reach the desired consistency. Serve the eggs on a warmed plate.

> TIP: Add ½ cup of your choice of chopped veggies along with an additional sprinkle of cheese and fold the eggs over to enjoy as an omelet.

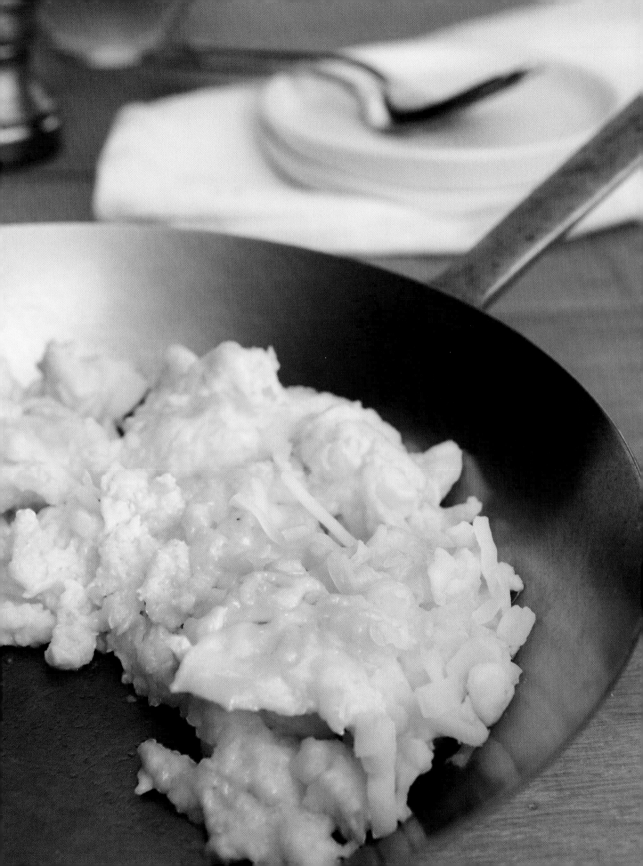

Castrofilippo Breakfast

This recipe is similar to what I used to eat for breakfast as a child growing up in Castrofilippo. I would take a tin cup to the woman down the road, and she'd skim off some ricotta for me from the whey of the sheep's milk she'd collected that morning. Then I'd run home, and my mother would prepare the rest. Nowadays, I simulate the recipe as best I can in New York City and still love it.

You'll notice the recipe calls for day-old bread. Bread was such an important part of our diet that it was never wasted. Once past its prime—which happens very quickly—it was repurposed for everything from the bread crumbs sprinkled over pasta to slices placed at the bottom of soup or under fish to add substance. In Italy they don't consider it stale; they call it *pane raffermo,* meaning "firmed-up bread." For this dish, you can use any kind of bread you like, but I prefer slices of day-old Italian baguette.

SERVES 1

2 slices day-old bread, broken up into 1-inch pieces (see Tip)

¼ cup milk

¼ cup hot coffee

¼ to ½ cup ricotta cheese

1 teaspoon sugar

1. Place the broken-up bread into a bowl. Warm the milk in a small pot over medium heat (do not boil) and pour it over the bread, along with the hot coffee. It will quickly soak into the bread and create a very soft consistency.

2. Scoop the ricotta cheese onto the top, stir it into the bread mixture, and sprinkle sugar on top. If the ricotta seems cold, you may want to put it in the microwave for 20 seconds before serving.

> TIP: Here are some other ways to make use of day-old crusty bread: grate it or send it for a few whirls in the food processor and use it for bread crumbs; toast cubes drizzled with olive oil at 400°F to make croutons; or enjoy it with one of my bruschetta recipes (pages 188–189).

Smoothies

Ⓚ kids

As you're probably aware, smoothies are thick and creamy drinks prepared in a blender. I always include fruit in my smoothies—you can experiment with different types and mix to taste. I prefer to use fresh fruit, but frozen fruits give the smoothie more of a milk-shake feel (adding crushed ice to fresh fruit will do this too). Bananas give smoothies a nice, dense, velvety consistency; you can use fresh or frozen, but frozen will be less fibrous and creamier. A little raw agave nectar, honey (for one year and up), or juice can be added to any smoothie to sweeten it up. I like to add a tablespoon of chopped fresh mint—it's delicious with any flavor of smoothie. Turn the page for some terrific variations to try.

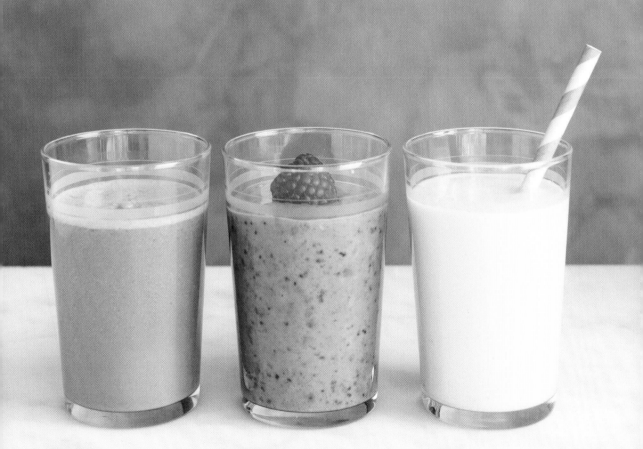

Fruit Smoothies with Almond Milk

SERVES 1 ADULT OR 2 CHILDREN

VERY BERRY

1 cup almond milk

½ cup blueberries

½ cup raspberries

1 banana

KIWI SURPRISE

1 cup almond milk

½ cup blueberries

½ cup raspberries

1 banana

2 kiwifruit

1 tablespoon chopped fresh mint leaves, optional

ANTIOXIDANT BLAST

1 cup almond milk

½ cup spinach leaves

½ cup kale leaves

3 ounces frozen mango (about ⅔ cup)

⅔ cup banana (fresh or frozen, better if frozen)

1 teaspoon honey (for 1 year and up) or raw agave nectar

In a blender, combine the ingredients for your chosen smoothie and puree until smooth.

> TIP: Puree a vegetable you'd like to use up and add it to a fruit smoothie (or try a veggie smoothie!).

Yogurt Smoothies

Don't worry if you have leftovers—I always like to make more than anyone will drink because you can leave it in the fridge and people will snack on it.

SERVES 1 ADULT OR 2 CHILDREN

TRIPLE BERRY
¼ cup raspberries
¼ cup blueberries
¼ cup blackberries
½ frozen banana

½ cup plain unsweetened
    Greek yogurt
1 tablespoon honey (for 1 year
    and up), optional

TROPICAL DELIGHT
1 frozen banana
½ cup frozen pineapple
½ cup mango pieces
½ cup plain unsweetened Greek
    yogurt

¼ cup juice (such as orange or
    pineapple)

In a blender, combine the ingredients for your chosen smoothie and puree until smooth.

Nut Butter Smoothie

SERVES 1 ADULT OR 2 CHILDREN

2 tablespoons peanut, almond,
    or sunflower seed butter
½ cup blueberries, raspberries,
    or blackberries

1 banana
1 cup almond milk
1 tablespoon honey (for 1 year
    and up), optional

In a blender, combine the ingredients and puree until smooth.

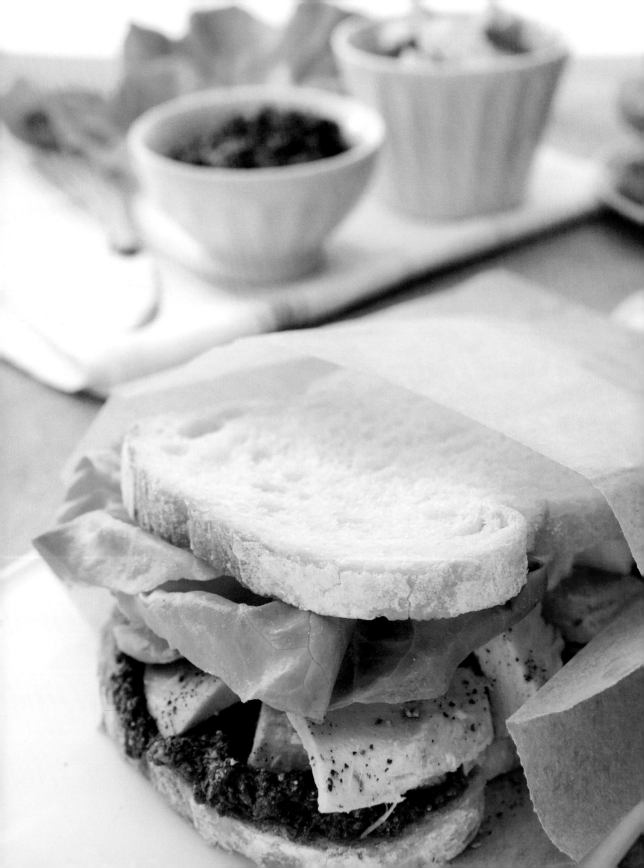

Super Quick Lunches

Here are a few ideas using staples from the pantry and long-lasting produce you're likely to have on hand.

Canned Tuna Salad with Capers

SERVES 2 TO 4

2 (6-ounce) cans tuna packed
   in oil, drained (preferably an
   Italian brand)
½ tablespoon Dijon mustard
2 tablespoons capers, chopped
½ medium onion, chopped
Juice of 1 lemon

3 cornichons, chopped
1 tablespoon mayonnaise
1 stalk celery, finely chopped
½ teaspoon salt
1 teaspoon black pepper
3 tablespoons extra-virgin olive
   oil

Combine the tuna, mustard, capers, onion, lemon juice, cornichons, mayo, and celery in a bowl. Sprinkle with salt and pepper, add the olive oil, mix again, and serve. You can eat this plain, on a bed of lettuce, or make a sandwich out of it (add a couple leaves of lettuce like romaine and some tomato slices, and serve it on a ciabatta roll or Italian bread slices).

Bean Salad with Tuna

SERVES 4

2 (6-ounce) cans tuna packed
   in oil, drained (preferably an
   Italian brand)
2 (14- to 16-ounce) cans butter
   beans or cannellini beans,
   drained
½ medium onion, chopped
1 stalk celery, chopped
1 teaspoon fresh thyme,
   chopped

1 tablespoon fresh basil,
   chopped
½ teaspoon salt
1 teaspoon black pepper
Juice of 1 lemon
1 tablespoon red or white wine
   vinegar
3 tablespoons extra-virgin olive
   oil

continued >

Toss all the ingredients into a large bowl and mix well. I use butter beans for this recipe; they're bigger than cannellini beans and creamier, but may not be as easy to find. Either bean works very well.

Mackerel and Potato Salad

Canned mackerel is an easy way to get oily fish—and it's a small fish so it doesn't have the mercury but is very high in healthy omega-3 fats. It's twice as expensive as tuna but well worth it. This is a nice recipe for those who don't have fresh mackerel available.

SERVES 4

½ pound fingerling potatoes, washed
1½ teaspoons salt
3 (4-ounce) cans mackerel packed in oil, drained
15 Kalamata olives, pitted and halved

2 tablespoons capers
Juice of 1 lemon
¼ cup extra-virgin olive oil
1 tablespoon red wine vinegar
1 teaspoon black pepper

Place the potatoes in a pan filled with cold water; add 1 teaspoon of the salt, bring to a boil, and cook until they are fork-tender, 5 to 7 minutes. Drain and rinse them under cold running water. Cut the potatoes into ¼-inch slices, then combine them with the mackerel, olives, capers, lemon juice, oil, vinegar, the remaining ½ teaspoon salt, and the pepper. Mix well, breaking up the mackerel fillets into smaller pieces.

> TIP: If you have a fillet of sole or a chicken cutlet left over—or anything thin enough—you can make sandwiches out of it. I suggest adding a few arugula leaves and some bruschetta topping (see my bruschetta recipes on pages 188–189).

Purees

Ⓑ babies
Ⓚ kids
Ⓢ seniors

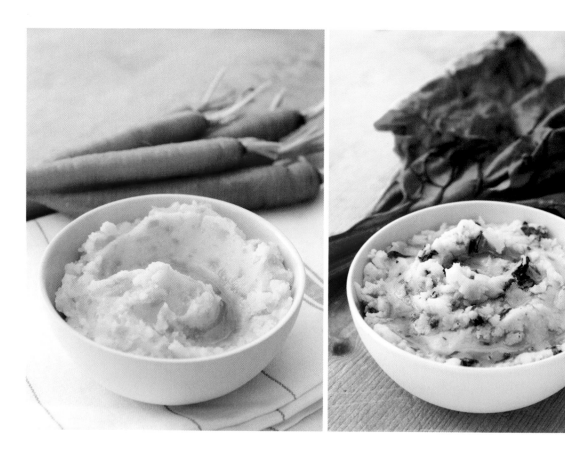

Vegetable Purees

B babies **K** kids

I don't include many purees for babies, because they can and should participate in the grown-up meals at the table—it's the Mediterranean way. You can turn most any recipe into a puree with a blender; my mother used to just mash things up with a fork. As I have explained, this establishes babies' preference for healthy foods. Of course, you have to be aware of a few particular precautions for infants, as well as your family's history of allergies. If there is a history, be sure to consult with your doctor as to what's appropriate for your child. The purees I include are here because they're also appealing to the adults at the table. In general, when sharing with babies, minimize salt and added sugar, and you might want to leave out strongly flavored spices. If you like, add spices and a little salt for the adults after the baby's portions have been set aside. The proportions make these purees easy to prepare for children's meals—just multiply depending on how many people are at the table.

NOTE: For any of the purees, you may add a little more olive oil to make them softer or adjust to your desired consistency. For a creamier consistency, add 2 tablespoons of cooking water or milk.

EACH VARIATION SERVES 2 ADULTS AS A SIDE DISH;
SERVINGS FOR CHILDREN VARY DEPENDING ON AGE OF CHILD

Swiss Chard

1 medium Idaho potato, peeled and quartered

3 leaves Swiss chard, stems removed, chopped

2 tablespoons extra-virgin olive oil

Pinch of salt, optional

1. Put the potato pieces in a small pot and add enough cold water to immerse them. Bring them to a boil and cook until the potato pieces are fork-tender, 8 to 10 minutes. Add the Swiss chard and cook for 4 to 5 minutes more.

2. Drain well, return the potato and chard to the pot, and combine the mixture well with a potato masher.

3. As you're mashing, add the olive oil (and salt for adults, if desired). Mash until you don't see whole leaves anymore but not until it's completely blended together.

Carrot

1 medium Idaho potato, peeled and quartered

¼ cup roughly chopped peeled carrot (about ½ carrot)

2 tablespoons extra-virgin olive oil

Pinch of salt, optional

1. Put the potato and carrot pieces in a small pot and add enough cold water to immerse them. Bring the water to a boil and cook until the vegetables are fork-tender, 8 to 10 minutes.

continued >

2. Drain well, return the potato and carrot to the pot, and combine them with a potato masher.

3. As you're mashing, add the olive oil (and salt for adults, if desired).

Spinach

1 medium Idaho potato, peeled and quartered	2 tablespoons extra-virgin olive oil
2 cups chopped stemmed fresh spinach or baby spinach	Pinch of salt, optional

1. Put the potato pieces in a small pot and add enough cold water to immerse them. Bring them to a boil and cook until the potato pieces are fork-tender, 8 to 10 minutes. Add the spinach and cook for 2 additional minutes.

2. Drain the vegetables well and return them to the pot. Add the olive oil (and salt for adults, if desired), and combine the mixture well with a potato masher. Mash until you don't see whole leaves anymore, but the mixture should not be completely blended together.

Pea

1 medium Idaho potato, peeled and quartered	2 tablespoons extra-virgin olive oil
¼ cup frozen peas	Pinch of salt, optional

1. Put the potato pieces in a small pot and add enough cold water to immerse them. Bring them to a boil and cook until the potato pieces are soft, 8 to 10 minutes (choose a shorter cooking time if the puree will be for adults only). Add the peas to the pot during the last 4 minutes of the cooking time, and continue to boil until the potato is done.

2. Drain the mixture well, return the potato and peas to the pot, and combine them with a potato masher.

3. As you're mashing, add the olive oil (and salt for adults, if desired).

Sweet Potato Puree

B babies **K** kids

The sweet potato is kind of a rock star among vegetables, chock-full of healthy ingredients like fiber, vitamins, and antioxidants. This makes it a go-to vegetable for kids, since they're naturally drawn to sweet. Leave the skins on to maximize the vegetable's nutrients if the children are old enough to eat it. To make it even more appealing to young palates, you can sprinkle a touch of brown sugar on top before you bake it, and it will melt into the potatoes.

SERVES 2 ADULTS AS A SIDE DISH; SERVINGS FOR CHILDREN VARY DEPENDING ON AGE OF CHILD

3 tablespoons extra-virgin olive oil

2 medium sweet potatoes, peeled and cut into ½-inch slices

½ teaspoon salt, optional

1. Preheat the oven to 425°F.

2. Oil a baking pan using 1 tablespoon of the olive oil, place the sliced potatoes on the sheet, and drizzle 1 tablespoon of the oil on top. Toss the potatoes to coat.

3. Sprinkle the potatoes with salt (if using), cover them with aluminum foil, and bake them for 30 to 40 minutes, until soft.

4. Transfer the baked potatoes to a bowl and mash them; mix in the remaining 1 tablespoon of oil with a fork.

QUICK TIP: If you're in a hurry, coat a whole sweet potato with a little olive oil, puncture it a few times with a fork, place it on a plate in the microwave, and cook on high for 5 to 10 minutes, flipping it over at the halfway point. You can then mash it or serve it as a baked potato.

Salads

Ⓑ babies
Ⓚ kids
Ⓢ seniors

Curly Kale Salad with Pine Nuts and Raisins

S seniors

SERVES 4

¼ cup extra-virgin olive oil

4 cloves garlic, crushed

2 bunches curly kale leaves,
    stems removed

3 tablespoons toasted pine nuts

3 tablespoons raisins

2 tablespoons balsamic vinegar

Salt and black pepper

1. In a small pan over low heat, combine the oil and garlic and heat them slowly. Do not allow to brown. Keep this warm while preparing the salad.

2. Finely chop the kale leaves julienne-style (long thin strips).

3. Strain out and discard the garlic from the warm oil. In a large bowl toss together the kale, pine nuts, raisins, balsamic vinegar, and garlic-flavored oil. The warm oil will help soften the kale.

4. Add salt and pepper to taste and serve.

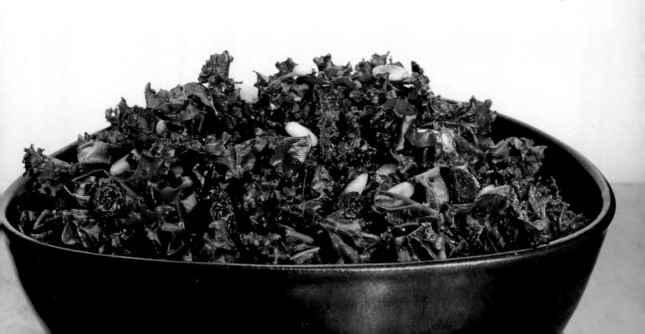

Mixed Salad alla Siciliana

Ⓢ seniors

This salad is typical of the Sicilian style, because we often threw whatever vegetables we had on hand—whatever was in season—into a salad. This might have included romaine lettuce, tomatoes, green beans, fava beans, and eggplant. We often picked the ingredients from our garden, mixed the salad, and ate it at a table we kept under a nearby walnut tree. All this is to say that, though the mix below tastes sensational, this recipe does not have to be exact. Use what you have available.

SERVES 6 TO 8

VINAIGRETTE

½ cup extra-virgin olive oil

⅓ cup lemon juice

1 tablespoon lemon zest

1 teaspoon salt

1 teaspoon black pepper

SALAD

1 head radicchio, roughly chopped (see Note)

1 head frisée lettuce, roughly chopped

1 head romaine lettuce, outer leavers removed, roughly chopped

1 fennel bulb, trimmed and thinly sliced

8 radishes, thinly sliced

½ cup asparagus, cut into 1-inch pieces

½ cup string beans, cut into 1-inch pieces

1 avocado, peeled and cut into 1-inch strips

Salt and black pepper

1. To prepare the vinaigrette, whisk together the oil, lemon juice and zest, salt, and pepper in a medium bowl and set aside. You can keep the dressing in the refrigerator for a couple of hours, if necessary (it's best used the same day it's prepared).

2. To make the salad, place the radicchio and lettuces in a large bowl and mix in the fennel and radish slices.

3. Bring a medium pot of water to a boil over high heat. Prepare a medium bowl of ice water and set it nearby. Blanch the asparagus and string beans in the boiling water for 4 minutes, then place them in the ice bath to stop the cooking process. Drain them well.

4. Add the asparagus and string beans to the lettuces along with the avocado. Toss in the vinaigrette, and add salt and pepper to taste.

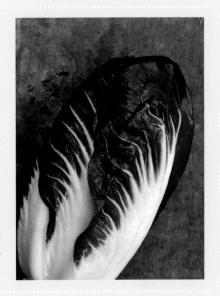

NOTE: I love using radicchio—a Mediterranean, maroon leafy vegetable with white veins, also known as Italian chicory. It's an excellent source of many vitamins (especially K), minerals, and antioxidants like lutein. It has a bitter and spicy taste, which mellows when it's grilled or roasted, but it's great fresh in salad. When choosing a head of radicchio, you want one that's firm and heavy. Radicchio doesn't spoil as quickly as many lettuces, which is a big plus.

VEGGIE-SAVING TIP: Chop up whatever leftover vegetables you have on hand, add a lettuce or two, and make a salad with them. Toss it with the vinaigrette from this recipe.

Insalata Palermitana

S seniors

Palermo is the capital of Sicily, and this is a typical salad from that city. Feel free to use any soft cheese for this recipe.

SERVES 4

DRESSING

1 tablespoon Dijon mustard

3 tablespoons sherry wine
   vinegar

1 teaspoon salt

1 teaspoon black pepper

¼ cup extra-virgin olive oil

SALAD

1 teaspoon salt

1 cup string beans, edges
   trimmed

8 fingerling potatoes, unpeeled,
   scrubbed

2 heads Bibb lettuce or hearts
   of romaine, leaves separated
   and washed and dried

4 plum tomatoes, sliced

¼ cup pitted Kalamata olives

¼ pound Fontina cheese, sliced
   into thin strips, or shredded

12 anchovy fillets

1. Bring a medium pot of water to a boil over high heat.

2. To prepare the dressing, put the mustard, vinegar, salt, and pepper in a bowl and mix with a fork. Slowly pour in the oil while continuing to whisk, until it is incorporated into the mixture, and set the dressing aside.

3. To prepare the salad, when the pot of water boils, add the salt and string beans. After the water returns to a boil, cook for another 2 minutes. Meanwhile, prepare a large bowl of ice water and set it nearby.

4. Remove the beans from the boiling water with a slotted spoon and place them in the ice water bath to stop the cooking process.

5. To the same pot of boiling water, add the potatoes and cook until they are fork-tender, 5 to 7 minutes. Drain and slice the potatoes into ¼-inch pieces.

6. Evenly divide the lettuce, string beans, potatoes, tomatoes, and olives among the serving plates. Top each salad with strips of cheese and 3 anchovy fillets and drizzle on the dressing just before serving.

Healthy Coleslaw

This dish is best after being chilled for twenty-four hours.

SERVES 6

3 bay leaves

1 tablespoon salt

¼ cup white vinegar

¼ cup extra-virgin olive oil

1 clove garlic, crushed

¼ cup sugar

1 medium cabbage, shredded (about 5 cups)

3 carrots, peeled and shredded

1. Place the bay leaves in a pot with 1 quart of cold water, bring the water to a boil, then allow the mixture to come to room temperature. Remove and discard the bay leaves.

2. Mix the salt, vinegar, oil, garlic, and sugar in a separate bowl; stir in the bay leaf–flavored water.

3. Place the cabbage and carrots into a large container with a lid. Slowly pour the marinade into the cabbage mixture, press it gently, cover it with the lid, and place the slaw in the refrigerator. The longer it chills, the better it tastes, so leave it for at least 2 hours (and up to 24). Remove the garlic before serving.

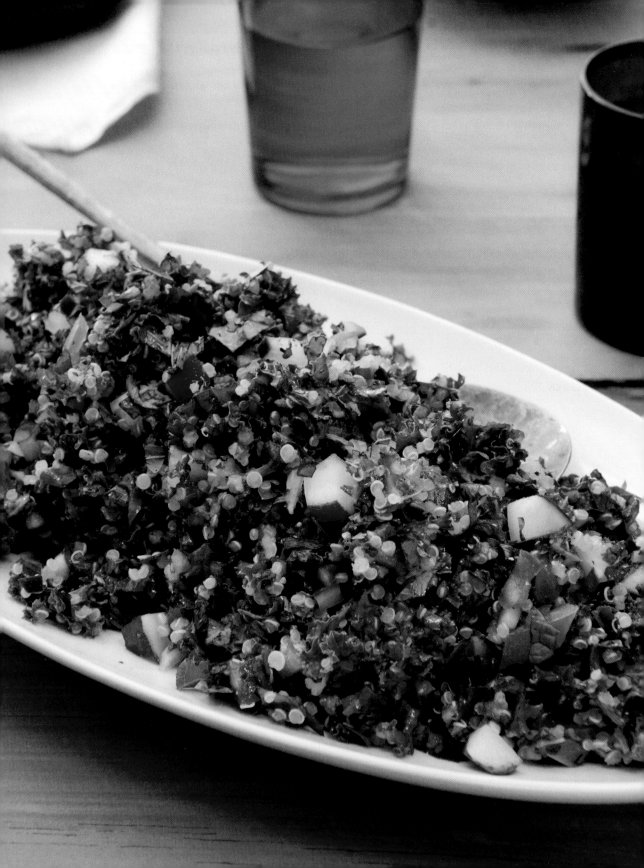

Tabbouleh Salad with Quinoa

Quinoa is a gluten-free source of protein, iron, and fiber.

SERVES 4

TABBOULEH

1 cup quinoa, rinsed

1 bunch kale leaves, stems
   removed, leaves finely
   chopped (see Note)

½ cup seeded, chopped plum
   tomatoes

⅓ cup finely chopped cucumber

½ cup finely chopped parsley

¼ cup chopped radishes

1 tablespoon chopped fresh mint

DRESSING

¼ cup extra-virgin olive oil

Juice of 1½ lemons

1 teaspoon salt

1 teaspoon black pepper

½ teaspoon ground cumin

1. Combine the quinoa with 1¾ cups water in a medium pot, and bring the mixture to a boil over high heat.

2. Lower the heat, cover the pot, and simmer the quinoa for 20 to 25 minutes, until the liquid is absorbed.

3. Remove from the heat and fluff with a fork. Allow to cool to room temperature.

4. Toss the cooked quinoa into a large bowl with the kale, tomatoes, cucumber, parsley, radishes, and mint.

5. To make the dressing, in a smaller bowl, whisk together the oil and lemon juice; add the salt, pepper, and cumin, and mix well.

6. Add the dressing to the salad and toss.

> **NOTE:** Kale is rich in calcium and vitamin K, known to ward off osteoporosis and strengthen bones, respectively.

Fennel and Orange Salad

This is a favorite of mine from Sicily. It's best served chilled.

SERVES 4

3 fennel bulbs, fronds removed
½ cup pomegranate seeds
1 medium-size red onion, thinly sliced
2 oranges, peeled, with segments separated and cut in half

¼ cup freshly squeezed orange juice
2 tablespoons lemon juice
1 teaspoon salt
1 teaspoon black pepper
4 tablespoons extra-virgin olive oil

1. Remove and discard the outer tough husks from the fennel bulbs. Halve each bulb and thinly slice it, ideally with a mandoline.

2. Combine the fennel, pomegranate seeds, onion, and orange in a large bowl. Refrigerate the mixture for 30 minutes.

3. In a separate bowl, combine the orange juice, lemon juice, salt, and pepper. Whisk in the oil and dress the salad.

The Surprising Healthfulness of Oranges

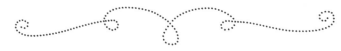

While citrus groves are plentiful in Sicily and thus the fruits are often included in recipes from the region, I'd like to highlight the particularly healthful qualities of the orange. An orange has more than 170 different phytonutrients and more than 60 flavonoids, many of which have been shown to have anti-inflammatory, antitumor, and blood-clot-inhibiting properties, as well as strong antioxidant effects. Among its many virtues, the orange . . .

- Is low-glycemic, so it doesn't make your blood sugar spike.

- Is abundant in cancer-fighting limonoids, which also help prevent kidney stones.
- Contains soluble fiber, which helps keep you full, and lowers your cholesterol.
- Possesses abundant polyphenols, which may protect against viral infections.
- Includes carotenoid compounds, which get converted to vitamin A and help prevent vision loss from macular degeneration.
- Is full of beta-carotene, a powerful antioxidant that protects the skin from free radicals and thus helps prevent the signs of aging.

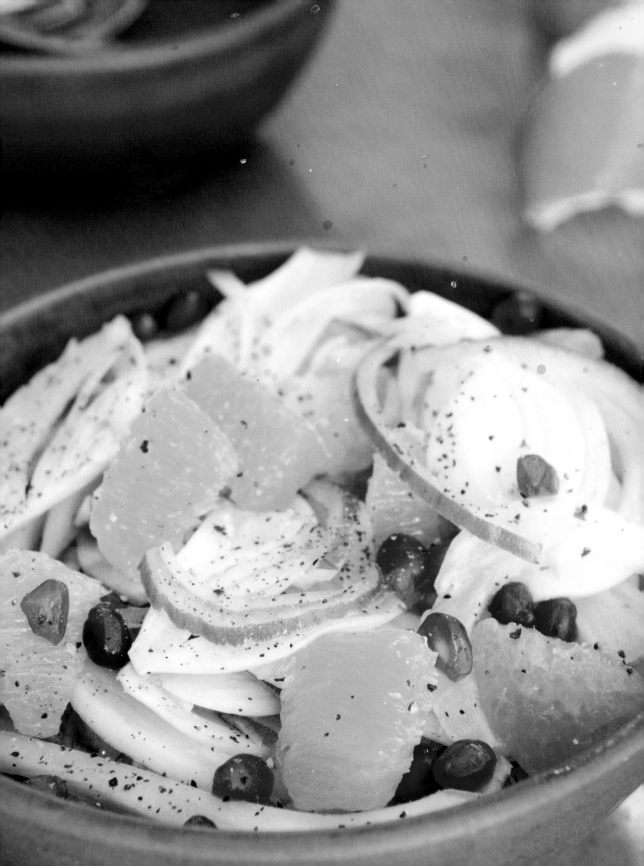

Salad with Grilled Chicken and Capers

SERVES 4

6 tablespoons extra-virgin olive
  oil
3 tablespoons red wine vinegar
1 teaspoon salt
1 teaspoon black pepper
4 heaping tablespoons capers,
  drained

1 head romaine lettuce, outer
  leaves removed, inner leaves
  chopped and chilled
2 freshly grilled chicken breasts,
  cut into bite-size pieces

1. In a small bowl, whisk the oil and vinegar together, then add the salt, pepper, and capers.

2. Combine the lettuce and chicken breast pieces in a large bowl.

3. Add the salad dressing to the salad bowl. Toss well and serve while the chicken is still warm.

> TIP: Most salad greens with vegetables taste great when chilled. When you have the time, plan to cover undressed salad greens and vegetables with plastic wrap and put it in the fridge for 30 minutes to 1 hour before serving.

Chickpea and Tuna Salad

This recipe can also be prepared with grilled fresh tuna, shrimp, or scallops.

SERVES 4

2 (6-ounce) cans chunk tuna in oil, drained

2 (14- to 16-ounce) cans chickpeas, drained

1 red onion, chopped

2 fresh plum tomatoes, seeded and chopped

2 tablespoons chopped fresh parsley

2 tablespoons chopped fresh basil

¼ cup extra-virgin olive oil

1 teaspoon red wine vinegar

Juice of 1½ lemons

1 teaspoon salt

1 teaspoon black pepper

1. Place the tuna in a large bowl and crumble it slightly with a fork.

2. Add the chickpeas, onion, tomatoes, parsley, basil, oil, vinegar, lemon juice, salt, and pepper.

3. Mix well and serve.

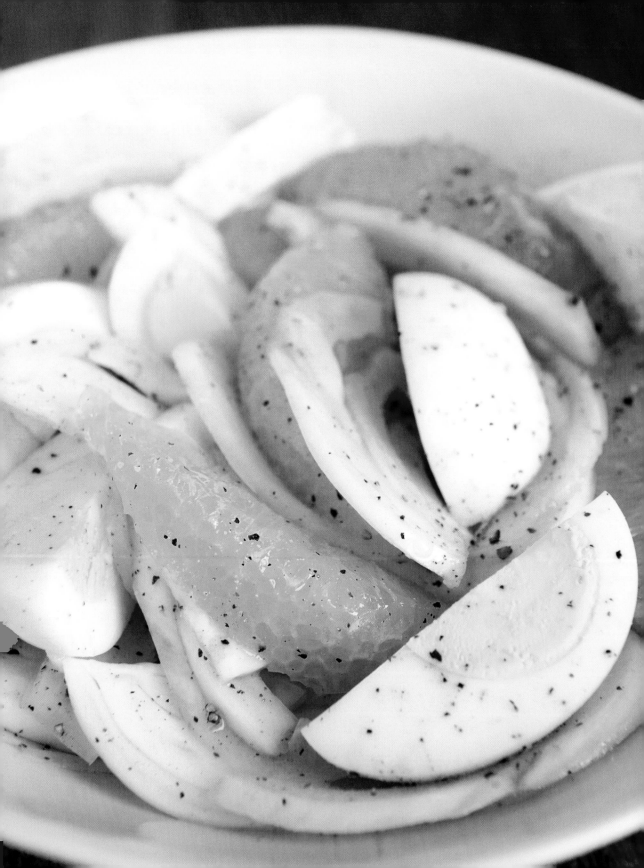

Orange and Egg Salad

K kids **S** seniors

You may think that this dish sounds strange. Everyone thinks so until they taste it! I often serve this salad with a slice of Italian baguette. It is also delicious without the fennel, if you don't have that available.

SERVES 4

4 hard-boiled eggs (see Note)
1 fennel bulb, fronds removed
  and outer husk trimmed away,
  thinly sliced
2 oranges, peeled and divided
  into segments

3 tablespoons extra-virgin olive
  oil
½ teaspoon salt
1 teaspoon black pepper

1. Peel the eggs and cut them into quarters. Place them in a large, low-rimmed bowl.

2. Add the fennel, oranges, oil, salt, and pepper, and mix gently.

NOTE: To get perfectly cooked and easy-to-peel hard-boiled eggs, put the eggs in a pot large enough to hold them all without touching and add enough cold water to cover them. Bring the water to a boil, then immediately shut off the heat. Allow the eggs to stand in the water for 5 minutes. Then remove them from the water carefully, peel them, and serve them or use them for your recipe.

Broiled Eggplant and Tomato Salad

S seniors

SERVES 4

SALAD

4 baby eggplants, partially
   peeled (run a peeler from top
   to bottom 3 times, making
   stripes), cut into 1-inch cubes
3 tablespoons extra-virgin
   olive oil

1½ teaspoons salt
1 pint cherry tomatoes, cut in
   half
2 tablespoons roughly chopped
   fresh basil

DRESSING

½ cup extra-virgin olive oil
2 cloves garlic, finely chopped
2 tablespoons red or white wine
   vinegar

1 teaspoon black pepper
½ teaspoon salt

1. To prepare the salad, set the oven to broil.

2. Place the eggplant cubes on a nonstick baking pan in a single layer. Coat them and toss with the oil and sprinkle with the salt.

3. Broil them for 5 to 7 minutes, tossing them a couple of times, until they are golden.

4. Place the broiled eggplant into a large bowl. Add the tomatoes and basil.

5. For the dressing, in a bowl, whisk together the oil, garlic, vinegar, pepper, and salt. Pour the dressing over the salad and toss before serving.

> TIP: For large and/or older eggplants, salting the eggplant ahead of cooking will make it less spongy and give it better flavor (it's not necessary for smaller, young ones). Salt will draw out liquid, making the eggplant more firm and expelling the seeds' bitter liquid. Salting also lowers the amount of oil needed because it won't absorb into the eggplant as much. Season the cut-up eggplant generously with coarse salt and let sit for 20 minutes to an hour, then rinse off the salt with cold water and pat dry. Reduce salt in the recipe by half if this is not taken into account already (my recipes assume you have not pre-salted).

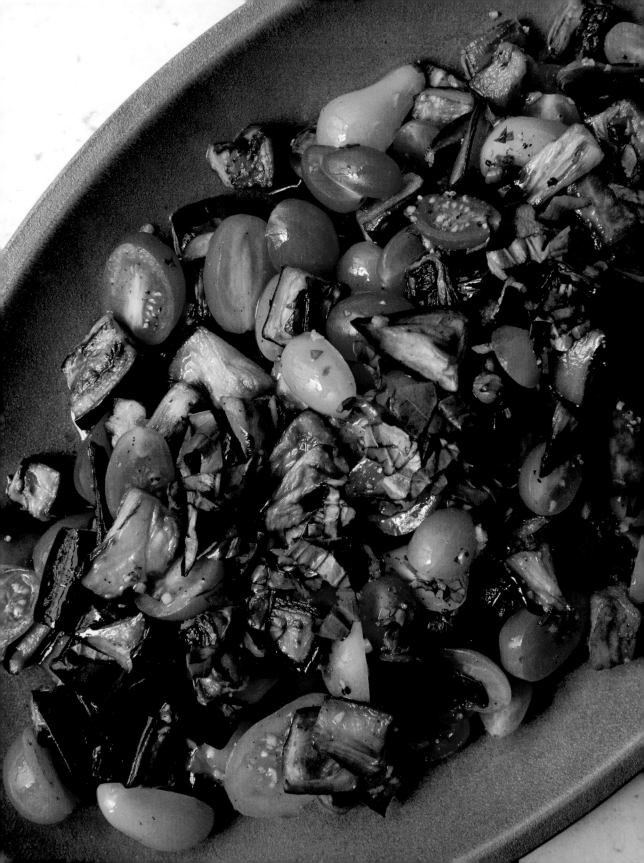

Orange and Olive Salad

This salad showcases the natural bounty of oranges and olives found in Sicily. It offers a perfect balance of sweet and salty. I call for green olives, but you can use any favorite type that you may have.

SERVES 4

6 oranges
1 cup pitted green olives, sliced
   in half

½ teaspoon black pepper
¼ teaspoon salt
¼ cup extra-virgin olive oil

1. Peel the oranges, removing as much of the pith (the white part) as possible. Cut the oranges in half, and slice them into half-moons ⅓ inch thick.

2. Add the oranges to a large bowl and mix in the olives, pepper, and salt. Drizzle with the oil and toss well.

Mediterranean Potato Salad

This recipe is typical of what my mother would make in Sicily. It's best enjoyed when the potatoes are still warm. I like to make it with white balsamic vinegar, which is unfamiliar to many. It has a sweet, pungent taste—without the acidity of red or white wine vinegar. The white balsamic makes a big difference and tastes wonderful.

SERVES 4

4 Yukon Gold potatoes, peeled and cut into 2-inch cubes
1½ teaspoons salt
2 tablespoons white balsamic vinegar (or use red or white wine vinegar)

½ teaspoon black pepper
1 clove garlic, minced
½ teaspoon dried oregano
6 tablespoons extra-virgin olive oil

1. Add the potatoes and 1 teaspoon of the salt to a large pot of cold water. Bring them to a boil over high heat and cook until they are fork-tender, about 10 minutes.

2. Meanwhile, in a small bowl, combine the vinegar, pepper, garlic, oregano, and the remaining ½ teaspoon salt. Whisk in the oil.

3. Drain the potatoes and put them into a large serving bowl. Add the dressing and toss to combine.

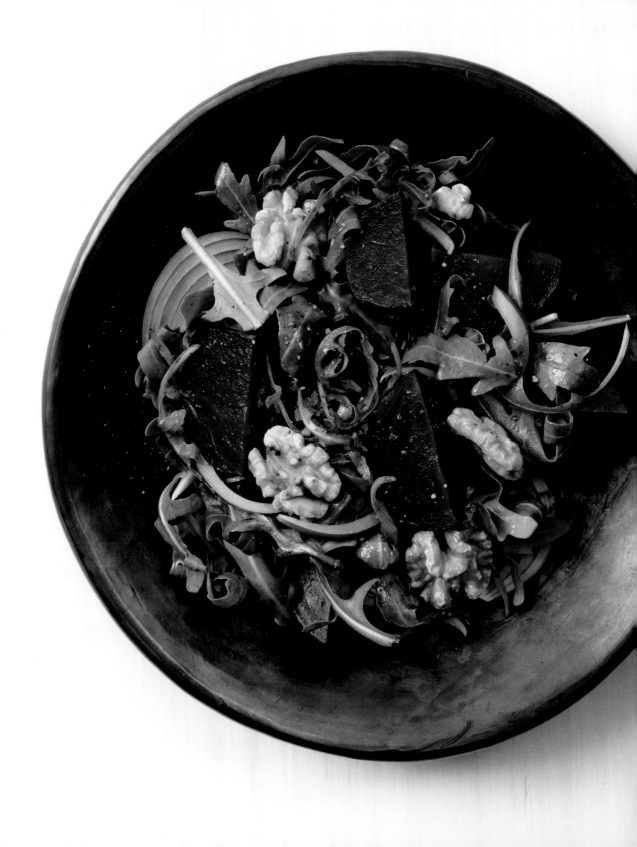

Balsamic Roasted Beet Salad

This is a very healthy salad with many elements of the Mediterranean diet, including antioxidant-rich veggies and omega-3-loaded nuts.

SERVES 6

1 tablespoon Dijon mustard
3 tablespoons balsamic vinegar
1 teaspoon salt
1 teaspoon black pepper
6 tablespoons extra-virgin olive
   oil

6 raw medium beets
½ red onion, sliced
1 handful almonds or walnuts
2 bunches arugula, washed and
   dried

1. Preheat the oven to 450°F.

2. In a small bowl, combine the mustard, vinegar, salt, and pepper. Slowly whisk in the oil, then set the vinaigrette aside.

3. Wrap the beets in a sheet of aluminum foil and bake them for 45 minutes to 1 hour (until the beets are fork-tender or soft enough to allow you to put a knife through them).

4. Allow the beets to cool, then peel and slice them into wedges.

5. Place the beets in a bowl, add the onion, pour half of the vinaigrette over the vegetables, and toss.

6. Place a dry pan over medium heat, then add the nuts and toast them for 2 to 3 minutes, tossing regularly to prevent burning.

7. Place the arugula into a bowl and dress it with the remainder of the vinaigrette.

8. For each serving plate, create a bed of arugula and top it with some of the beet mixture and then a sprinkling of nuts.

TIP: If you'd like, add crumbled blue cheese to this salad—it tastes great.

Insalata Comisana
(Salad with Pecorino Cheese)

Comisana is a breed of sheep in Sicily, and pecorino is made with sheep's milk. Today cow's milk cheese is more familiar, but pecorino was one of the most common kinds of cheese around when I was growing up, because we had few cows. You can make this salad with any kind of lettuce—I prefer butter leaf or romaine.

SERVES 4

2 oranges

1 fennel bulb, fronds and outer husk trimmed, quartered and thinly sliced

6 lettuce leaves, cut into strips

1 green apple, peeled, cored, and cut into chunks

1 medium red onion, thinly sliced

3 tablespoons extra-virgin olive oil

½ teaspoon salt

1 tablespoon balsamic vinegar

¼ teaspoon red pepper flakes

½ cup shaved pecorino cheese

1. Peel the oranges, removing as much of the pith (the white part) as possible, separate them into sections, and cut the orange wedges in two.

2. Put the oranges, fennel, lettuce, apple, and onion in a large bowl. Drizzle the oil over all, then sprinkle on the salt, vinegar, and red pepper flakes; toss the salad. Serve it with the shaved cheese on top.

Mushroom Salad

You can prepare this salad with all white button mushrooms if you don't have cremini.

SERVES 4

½ pound white button mushrooms, stemmed and thinly sliced

½ pound cremini mushrooms, stems removed, thinly sliced

3 inner stalks celery, thinly sliced

Juice of 1 lemon

½ teaspoon salt

½ teaspoon black pepper

¼ cup extra-virgin olive oil

1 tablespoon chopped fresh parsley

½ cup shaved Parmigiano cheese

1. Place the mushrooms and celery in a large bowl.

2. In a small bowl, combine the lemon juice, salt, and pepper. Slowly whisk in the olive oil.

3. Toss the mushrooms and celery with the dressing, then mix in the parsley.

4. Place the salad on individual serving plates and top each portion with shaved Parmigiano cheese.

Whitefish Salad

My father absolutely loved this salad. I used to buy it for him at an Italian specialty store, and when I had the time to make it for him myself, he liked my variation even more. The store-bought version had a little mayonnaise, salt, and pepper, and that was it. I add a bit of flavor to give it a kick.

SERVES 4 TO 6

1 medium smoked whitefish
1 tablespoon mayonnaise
3 tablespoons plain Greek yogurt
3 tablespoons capers, chopped
3 stalks celery, finely chopped
½ medium onion, finely chopped

½ teaspoon salt
1 teaspoon black pepper
Juice of ½ lemon
2 tablespoons extra-virgin olive
  oil

1. Remove the meat from the bones of the fish, place it in a medium bowl, and break it up into 1-inch pieces with your hands.

2. In a separate medium bowl, use a fork to mix the mayonnaise and yogurt.

3. Mix in the capers, celery, onion, salt, pepper, lemon juice, and oil. Stir in the whitefish meat and serve. This salad will keep in the fridge for up to two days.

Soups

Ⓑ   babies

Ⓚ   kids

Ⓢ   seniors

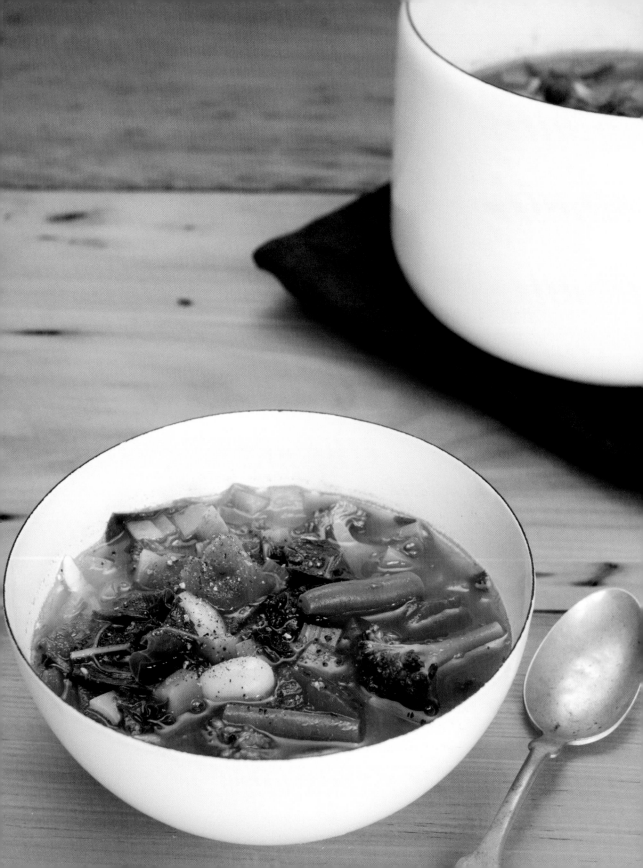

Minestrone Soup, Three Ways

K kids **S** seniors

Minestrone soup doesn't have to have a strict recipe. I offer three suggestions here, but you can add vegetables according to your taste and what you have on hand. Our minestrone soup was always changing in Sicily depending on what vegetables were in season. Whatever vegetables were left over got thrown in the pot.

We always make more of these soups than we can eat. Whatever's left we put in the fridge and have as a snack or with a meal over the next few days, or we freeze it for later.

For babies, you can puree these soups for a smoother consistency. As all of these minestrone soups contain tomatoes, if your baby is under one year of age, ask your doctor when it's safe for him or her to begin eating tomatoes.

Minestrone Soup with Kale

This is a terrific recipe for so many reasons. It's easy, fast, and you can make it all in one pot. My wife loves it when I make this because I make a giant pot for dinner together with our children. When our little ones were very young, starting at around nine months old, my wife and I would eat the soup as prepared, and then put it in the blender and puree it for them. (See the Tip on page 152.) We would include orzo to make the soup more substantial, adding it before or after the blending so there were options for different ages. It's also easy to tailor the vegetable combination to your taste and your children's. For example, one of my boys never took a liking to peas; he would always reject them if they weren't blended in so he couldn't spot them. So we would make minestrone with cannellini beans—a slightly different flavor, and just as delicious. The variation here includes kale—native to the Mediterranean region and a member of the broccoli and cauliflower family—which has remarkably high levels of antioxidants, as well as vitamins, minerals, calcium, potassium, protein, and fiber.

6 tablespoons extra-virgin olive oil

1 (14-ounce) can crushed
  tomatoes

1 tablespoon salt, optional

2 carrots, cut into ¼-inch cubes

1 medium onion, chopped

½ head broccoli, cut into 1-inch
  florets (2 to 3 cups, the more
  the better)

1 leek, white part only, chopped

2 stalks celery, cut into ¼-inch
  cubes

2 cups chopped kale leaves

1 cup string beans, ends trimmed,
  cut into 1-inch pieces

1 (8-ounce) can chopped tomatoes

2 (14-ounce) cans cannellini
  beans, drained and rinsed, or
  2 cups frozen peas, defrosted

1 cup short pasta such as tubetti
  for adults or orzo for kids,
  cooked according to package
  instructions, optional

Black pepper, optional

1. In a large pot over low heat, heat 1 tablespoon of the olive oil and cook the tomatoes for 15 minutes.

2. Add 2 quarts of water and bring it to a boil; add salt (if desired), 1 tablespoon of the oil, and the carrots, onion, broccoli, leek, celery, kale, string beans, and tomatoes.

3. Bring the soup to a boil, then reduce the heat and simmer it for 20 to 25 minutes, adding the beans and pasta (if desired) during the last 5 minutes of cooking.

4. Use the remaining 4 tablespoons of oil to drizzle over the individual bowls (and add pepper to taste for adults, if desired).

> TIP: A convenient way to feed a baby with this dish is to puree it in the blender and then pour it into a tray of small plastic baby food containers or a flexible ice cube tray and freeze. You can defrost them as needed! Freeze the soup without pasta in it and add that after it's been thawed, if desired.

Chickpea Minestrone

The chickpeas and pasta in this minestrone make for a hearty spoonful.

SERVES 6 TO 8

1⅔ cups dried chickpeas, soaked overnight, or 4 (14-ounce) cans, drained and rinsed

1 teaspoon baking soda

1 tablespoon plus ½ teaspoon salt

7 tablespoons extra-virgin olive oil

1 large onion, chopped

3 plum tomatoes, peeled, seeded, and chopped

1 teaspoon chopped fresh rosemary

1 teaspoon black pepper

1 teaspoon red pepper flakes

½ cup ditalini pasta (or any short pasta you can eat with a spoon), cooked according to package instructions

1. If you're using dried chickpeas, drain the soaking water and rinse them. Place them in a large pot with enough water to cover them by two finger-widths. Add the baking soda and 1 teaspoon of the salt. Bring the water to a boil over high heat, lower the heat, and simmer until the chickpeas are cooked, 40 to 60 minutes. If you are using canned chickpeas, add enough water to cover them by two finger-widths, bring to a boil, and proceed as directed below.

2. In a separate pan, heat 4 tablespoons of the oil over medium heat, then add the onion, tomatoes, rosemary, black pepper, and red pepper flakes. Cook the mixture for 10 minutes, then add it to the cooked chickpeas in their water. If you are using canned chickpeas, add them to the mixture.

3. Remove the pot from the heat and allow it to sit for 5 minutes before serving to let the flavors mingle. Stir the ditalini into the minestrone just before serving. Use the remaining olive oil to drizzle over individual bowls.

On Cooking with Dried Beans

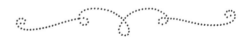

Some recipes call for dried beans, and some for canned; you can choose either. Cooked dried beans have a better texture than canned (they're not as mushy); they have retained more vitamins and minerals; and they don't contain the sodium added during the canning process. Canned beans are fine to use as a convenient option, though, and rinsing them before use will reduce their sodium content.

Four-Bean Minestrone with Rice

1 cup long-grain rice

⅔ cup extra-virgin olive oil

1 cup ½-inch-diced Idaho or
   Yukon Gold potatoes

1 medium onion, chopped

¼ cup chopped celery

½ cup chopped carrots

3 plum tomatoes, peeled and
   chopped

1 cup string beans, trimmed and
   cut into 1-inch pieces

1½ tablespoons salt

1 cup frozen peas

1 (14-ounce) can red kidney
   beans, drained and rinsed

1 (14-ounce) can cannellini
   beans, drained and rinsed

1 cup frozen fava beans, rinsed
   in cold water

½ cup grated Parmigiano cheese

1. Add the rice and 2 cups of water to a medium pot. Cover the pot, bring it to a boil, and then lower the heat to a simmer for 7 to 10 minutes, until the rice is tender. Set aside.

2. Add half of the oil to a large pot over medium-high heat and sauté the potatoes for 3 to 4 minutes, stirring frequently.

3. Add the onion, celery, and carrots to the pot. Sauté for 3 to 4 minutes and add the tomatoes. Cook for 2 to 3 minutes longer.

4. Add enough water to cover the vegetables by about two finger-breadths, bring the soup to a boil, and add the string beans and salt. Cook for 3 minutes.

5. Add the peas and the kidney, cannellini, and fava beans. Bring to a boil and cook for 2 to 3 minutes.

6. Add the rice until the soup is the desired consistency, along with the remaining oil, and stir to combine.

7. Sprinkle each serving with grated cheese.

Feast of San Giuseppe Bean Soup

B babies **K** kids **S** seniors

This soup was typically made in my hometown for the Feast of San Giuseppe. The original recipe calls for wild fennel, but here we will use the easier-to-find fennel fronds, or you can substitute dill.

The recipe is best prepared with dried legumes, not canned. You can choose from three different kinds of dried beans: lentils, cannellini beans, or kidney beans. If you choose the cannellini or kidney beans, you'll need to soak them overnight (but not the lentils). I prefer to use fresh tagliatelle pasta, which is similar to fettuccine but a little narrower and thinner. You can make it or buy it soft at the grocery store, or you can use the hard, dried version which is usually packaged in flat wrapped balls that resemble nests. The dried version cooks in about the same amount of time.

For babies, puree this soup for a smoother consistency.

SERVES 6

2 cups dried lentils, cannellini beans, or kidney beans (see page 152)
1 head broccoli, broken into large florets (about 3 cups)
2 cups chopped fennel or dill fronds

1 tablespoon salt, optional
1 tablespoon black pepper
8 ounces fresh tagliatelle, cut into 1-inch strips
¼ cup extra-virgin olive oil

1. If you are using either kidney or cannellini beans, place them in a large bowl with enough water to cover them, and let them soak overnight. Drain them just before proceeding.

2. Add the lentils or soaked beans to a large pot with the broccoli, fennel fronds, salt (if using), and pepper and add enough water to cover by two finger-widths. Cook the soup for 40 minutes over low heat. Add the tagliatelle and adjust the salt to taste. Cook for 5 minutes longer and serve with olive oil drizzled on top.

Leek and Cannellini Bean Soup

⑤ seniors

This soup is a terrific choice for those over sixty, as it's abundant in nutrients one especially needs later in life. These include healthy plant protein (older adults are prone to protein insufficiency), fiber, vitamin K, potassium, lysine to aid in calcium absorption, and folate to help reduce homocysteine levels, which are a major risk factor for heart disease. And of course, all soups are soft and so are a favorite for anyone with dental difficulties.

SERVES 4

½ cup extra-virgin olive oil
2 cups chopped leeks
1 cup chopped carrots
1 cup chopped celery
1 cup diced turnip
½ tablespoon salt

6 cups chicken stock or water
1½ (14- to 16-ounce) cans cannellini beans, drained and rinsed (about 2½ cups)
¼ cup grated Parmigiano cheese

1. In a large pot, put ¼ cup of the oil over high heat and heat until it shimmers. Add the leeks and sauté for 2 minutes.
2. Add the carrots, celery, turnip, and salt and cook for another 2 minutes. Add the chicken stock and bring the soup to a boil. Lower the heat, cover the pot, and simmer for 20 minutes.
3. Add the cannellini beans and simmer for another 2 minutes.
4. Ladle the soup into bowls. Sprinkle each portion with cheese and drizzle with a tablespoon of olive oil.

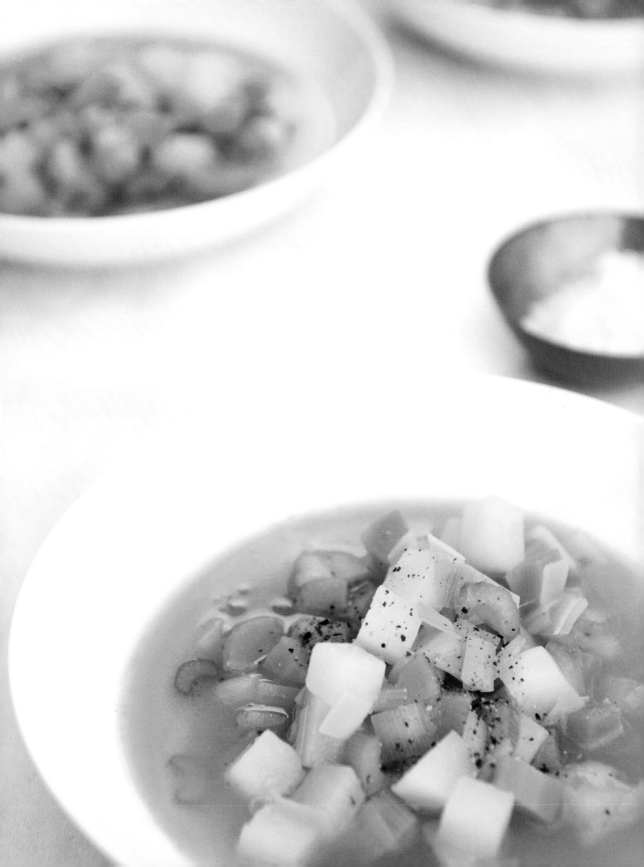

Chickpea and Spinach Soup

S seniors

This recipe comes from Massimo Carbone, a Sicilian chef at the restaurant Brio in Manhattan. I go to his restaurant to have this dish about once a week!

SERVES 4 TO 6

4 tablespoons extra-virgin olive oil

4 cloves garlic, crushed

1 tablespoon chopped rosemary

2 cups dried chickpeas, soaked overnight and drained, or 3 (14- to 16-ounce) cans chickpeas, drained and rinsed

1½ quarts vegetable broth or water

1 teaspoon salt

4 cups baby spinach

1. Put 2 tablespoons of the oil in a large pot over medium heat and add the garlic. Brown it for 1 to 1½ minutes to flavor the oil, then remove and discard the garlic.

2. Add the rosemary and chickpeas and sauté for 2 minutes. Add the vegetable broth and salt and bring the soup to a boil. Lower it to a simmer and cook it for 10 minutes if you're using canned chickpeas and 40 to 50 minutes if you're using soaked.

3. When the chickpeas are tender, remove 1 cup of them and liquefy them in a blender.

4. Return the pureed chickpeas to the pot, add the spinach, and cook for another minute.

5. Drizzle the soup with the remaining 2 tablespoons of oil prior to serving.

Hearty Soup

B babies **K** kids **S** seniors

For babies, this soup can be pureed into a smoother consistency.

SERVES 4

6 tablespoons extra-virgin olive
   oil
1 leek, white part only, chopped
2 carrots, cut into ¼-inch cubes
2 turnips, peeled and cut into
   ¼-inch cubes
1 teaspoon salt, optional

1 teaspoon black pepper
2 cups chopped Swiss chard
   leaves
1 (14-ounce) can cannellini
   beans, with its liquid
¼ cup grated Parmigiano cheese

1. Put 4 tablespoons of the olive oil in a medium pot over medium-high heat. Add the leek, carrots, zucchini, and turnips and sauté for 3 to 4 minutes.

2. Add the salt (if using) and pepper and enough water to cover the vegetables by 1 inch.

3. Bring the soup to a boil, cover the pot, and let it simmer over low to medium heat for 10 minutes.

4. Add the chard and cannellini beans and cook for another minute or two.

5. Ladle the soup into individual serving bowls, top with the cheese, and drizzle with the remaining 2 tablespoons of oil.

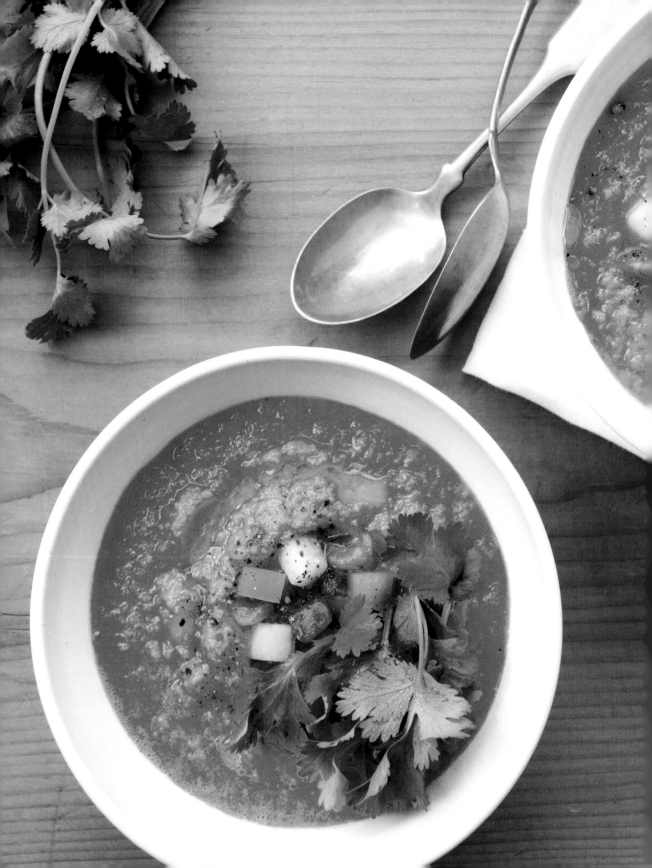

Gazpacho

Because this is a chilled soup, it's terrific in the summertime. All the ingredients in gazpacho should be finely chopped.

SERVES 4

6 plum tomatoes peeled, seeded, and finely chopped

2 cucumbers peeled, seeded, and finely chopped

1 medium onion, finely chopped

1 clove garlic, finely chopped

1 green pepper, finely chopped

2 tablespoons finely chopped fresh cilantro

2 tablespoons finely chopped fresh basil

2 jalapeño peppers, seeded and finely chopped

1½ teaspoons salt

1 teaspoon black pepper

4 tablespoons extra-virgin olive oil

2 cups tomato juice

1. In a large bowl, combine all the vegetables and herbs, the salt, black pepper, and 2 tablespoons of the olive oil; stir well. Set ¼ cup of this mixture aside.

2. Puree the remainder of the gazpacho mixture and the tomato juice in a blender. Put it in the refrigerator to chill for 30 to 45 minutes. To serve, top each bowl of gazpacho with 1 tablespoon of the reserved chopped vegetables and a drizzle of the remaining 2 tablespoons of oil.

Vegetables

Ⓑ babies
Ⓚ kids
Ⓢ seniors

Orange Winter Squash Sautéed with Garlic and Tomatoes

ⓢ seniors

Serve this hot with Italian bread for dunking.

SERVES 4

¼ cup extra-virgin olive oil
6 cloves garlic, crushed
⅔ cup crushed canned or
    roughly chopped fresh
    tomatoes
3 pounds winter squash such as
    calabaza, peeled, seeded, and
    cut into 2-inch cubes

½ tablespoon salt
8 leaves fresh basil, roughly
    chopped
½ teaspoon red pepper flakes

1. In a large pan over medium-high heat, add the olive oil and garlic and sauté until the garlic is golden.

2. Add the tomatoes, squash, salt, basil, red pepper flakes, and 1 cup of water. Bring the mixture to a boil.

3. Cover the pan and let the mixture simmer for 20 to 30 minutes, stirring every 5 minutes. The squash is cooked when it is fork-tender.

Carrots with Oregano and Vinegar

This dish will taste best after it sits for a long time at room temperature, which makes it perfect for meals served buffet-style or outside. Think family picnic.

SERVES 6

- 1 pound carrots, peeled and cut diagonally into thin, 2-inch-long slices
- 3 tablespoons extra-virgin olive oil
- 3 cloves garlic, crushed
- 1 teaspoon dry oregano
- 3 tablespoons red wine vinegar
- 1 teaspoon freshly ground black pepper
- 1 teaspoon salt

1. Place the carrots in a large pot of salted water over high heat. Bring to a boil and cook for 3 to 5 minutes, until fork-tender.

2. Drain the carrots well and place them in a deep serving bowl.

3. Add all the remaining ingredients and toss to coat.

4. Let the mixture sit for 4 to 6 hours and serve it at room temperature.

The Spices of Life: Adding Flavor Without Salt

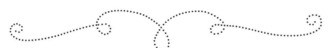

We tend to appreciate food more when our sense of taste is stimulated and surprised. When trying to cut down on unhealthful ingredients such as butter and salt, we might crave more flavor. Similarly, as we age, a drop in taste-bud power and saliva can leave some foods seeming more bland. Artfully flavoring food can compensate, but don't try to fix the problem by reaching for the salt shaker.

There are millions of wonderful seasonings that contain no sodium, or significantly less of it.

For example, add flavors you like such as black pepper, a splash of wine or lemon juice, red pepper flakes, poppy seeds, jalapeño, or salsa. Low-sodium soy sauce is another alternative. In savory cooking, use herbs, spices, garlic, and onion, like the Italians do, in place of salt or to minimize the need for salt, and avoid flavor-sapping overcooking. Try different food flavors and textures as well—you might find something new to stimulate your palate.

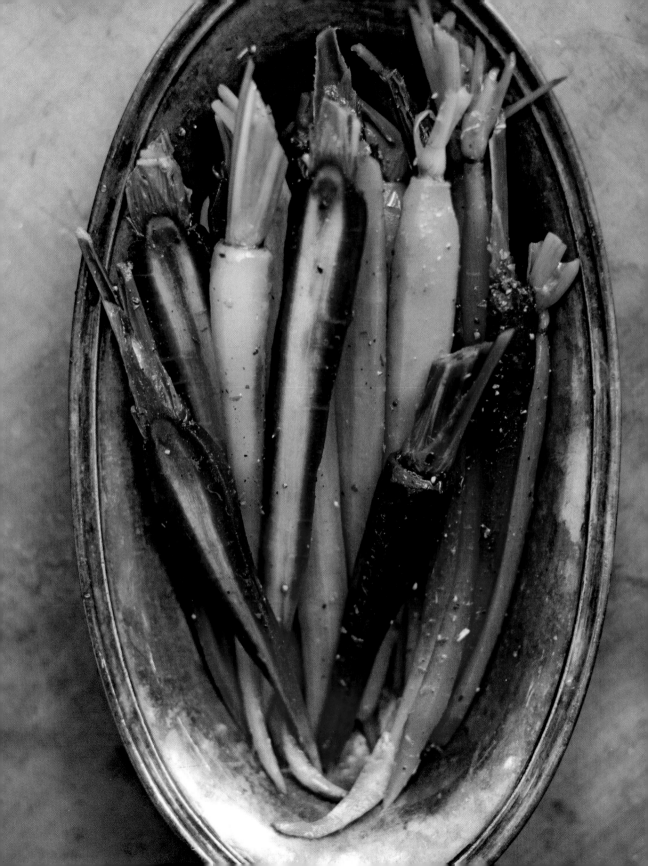

Roasted Broccoli with Parmigiano

This is a recipe of my mother's. As she's getting older, she appreciates recipes that are simpler to prepare and this is one of them. It's also a great dish for kids—you might say it's the healthy Mediterranean alternative to microwaving broccoli with a slice of American cheese on top!

SERVES 4

6 cups broccoli florets (a bit more than 1 head)

6 tablespoons extra-virgin olive oil

6 cloves garlic, sliced

½ tablespoon salt

1 teaspoon black pepper

1 tablespoon lemon juice

½ cup grated Parmigiano cheese

1. Preheat the oven to 400°F.

2. In a large bowl, mix the broccoli florets with 4 tablespoons of the olive oil, the garlic, salt, and pepper. Spread the florets on a baking pan in a single layer.

3. Bake them for 20 minutes.

4. Remove the broccoli from the oven and quickly, while it is still hot, drizzle it with the remaining 2 tablespoons of olive oil and the lemon juice. Sprinkle the Parmigiano over all.

Baked Butternut Squash with Onions and Brussels Sprouts

SERVES 6

4 pounds butternut squash, peeled, seeded, and cut into 3-inch wedges about 1 inch wide and ⅔ inch thick

10 tablespoons extra-virgin olive oil

1 teaspoon salt

1 teaspoon black pepper

4 large red onions, each cut into 8 wedges

1 pound Brussels sprouts, each cut in half

1. Preheat the oven to 400°F.

2. In a large bowl, mix the squash with 3 tablespoons of the oil and ½ teaspoon each of salt and pepper. Spread the squash on a baking pan in a single layer.

3. In the same large bowl, mix the onions and Brussels sprouts with 3 tablespoons of the oil and the remaining salt and pepper. Spread the vegetables on a separate baking pan in a single layer.

4. Add 3 tablespoons of water to each pan, cover them with foil, and place them in the oven.

5. Bake the onions and Brussels sprouts for 15 minutes. Uncover and cook them for another 7 to 10 minutes.

6. Bake the squash for 20 minutes. Uncover and cook it for another 10 minutes until it is fork-tender.

7. Combine the roasted vegetables in a large serving bowl and drizzle the remaining 4 tablespoons of oil over all.

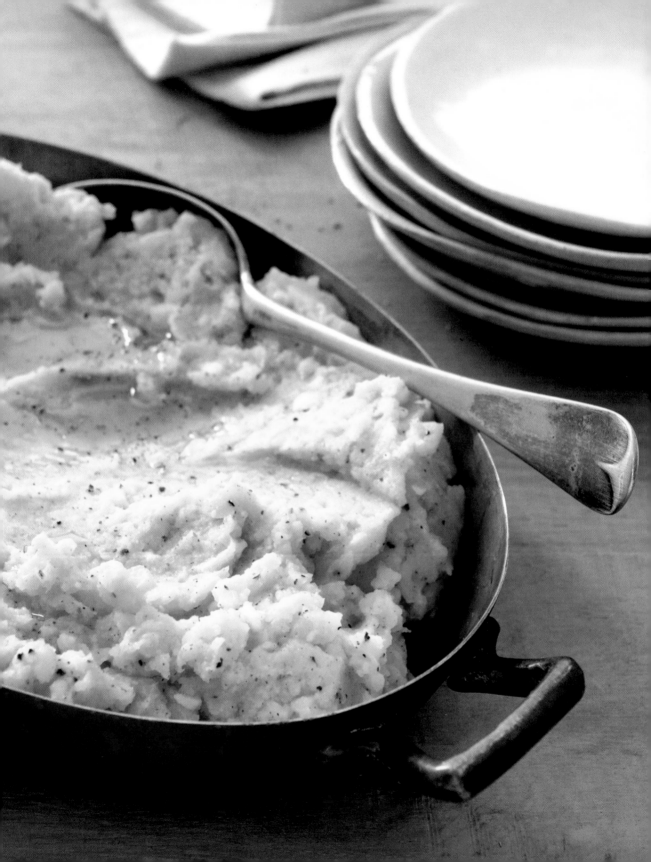

Olive Oil Mashed Potatoes

B babies K kids

Nix the butter-and-cream-loaded mashed potatoes and give this recipe a try. It's a great, versatile, go-to side, and it doesn't take any more time than the less nutritious version. I like to leave the potato skins on, because you get more vitamins, minerals, protein, and fiber that way. You can also prepare this dish with sweet potatoes to up the vitamin and mineral content even more.

SERVES 6

2 pounds Yukon Gold potatoes, peeled, if desired, and cut into 2-inch cubes
1 tablespoon salt
10 cloves garlic, peeled (use less—to taste—if for young children)

¼ cup extra-virgin olive oil
1 tablespoon black pepper

1. Place the potatoes, salt, and garlic in a large pot with enough water to cover. Place it over high heat and bring it to a boil. Cook until fork-tender, approximately 15 minutes.

2. Drain the garlic and potatoes, reserving approximately 1 cup of the cooking liquid.

3. Add the potatoes and garlic back to the pot and mash, adding the reserved water until you reach the desired consistency.

4. Add the oil and pepper slowly while vigorously stirring. Serve hot.

Stuffed Mushrooms with Spinach

SERVES 4

8 tablespoons extra-virgin olive
oil
½ cup plain bread crumbs
2 scallions, finely chopped
12 medium to large white button
mushrooms, caps kept whole,
stems removed and diced

1 teaspoon salt
1 teaspoon black pepper
4 cups baby spinach, roughly
chopped
2 tablespoons grated Parmigiano
cheese

1. Preheat the oven to 375°F.

2. Put 2 tablespoons of the oil in a pan over medium heat and toast the bread crumbs for approximately 2 minutes. Set them aside.

3. Put 2 tablespoons of the oil in a separate pan over medium-high heat and sauté the scallions.

4. After 2 minutes of cooking, add the chopped mushroom stems, salt, and pepper and cook for another 2 minutes.

5. Add the spinach and cook until it wilts, another minute or two.

6. Remove the pan from the heat, add the cheese, and stir well.

7. Grease a baking pan with 1 tablespoon of the oil and arrange the mushroom caps on the pan, cavity side up. Drizzle 1 tablespoon of oil evenly over the mushroom caps.

8. Stuff each mushroom with 1 teaspoon of the spinach mixture and top it with 1 teaspoon of the bread crumbs.

9. Use the remaining 2 tablespoons of oil to sprinkle the mushrooms, then bake them for 10 to 15 minutes.

Timing and Serving

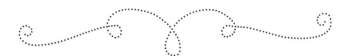

It's very important to get your timing down when cooking a meal so that you can serve your dishes at the appropriate temperatures. Many people don't pay attention to this detail, and it can really undermine all the effort you put into a meal.

The French have a term in cooking, *mise en place,* which means "everything in place." That is, before you cook, have everything as ready as possible—ingredients measured, peeled, and chopped; pans greased; tools and equipment within reach; and so on, as if you're ready to do your own cooking show. This will keep you from running around and burning your garlic while you're seasoning the halibut. The following tips will make your work in the kitchen more efficient and less stressful:

- Before you cook meat, chicken, or fish, take it out of the refrigerator for 30 minutes (don't forget to account for the time needed for this when you're planning your schedule).
- Prepare salads in advance, then place them in the refrigerator (just before you take them out, prepare the dressing).
- Prepare side dishes like vegetables before cooking the main dish.
- Use heat-resistant/oven-safe serving dishes so when something needs to be set aside and kept warm, such as side dishes or vegetables, you can place the dishes on turned-off hot burners or into a 175°F to 200°F oven (and not dirty another dish). You can keep premade dishes warming for up to 1 hour.
- You can cover many dishes with aluminum foil to retain warmth and prevent drying for up to 30 minutes. Fried foods, or any dishes with a crisp crust, should not be covered, as they will become soggy.
- Serve fish, pasta, and cuts of chicken immediately after cooking for the best flavor and texture. You can let roast chicken and meat rest (for about 15 minutes or 6 minutes, respectively) before cutting, as it gives the juices a chance to penetrate the meat.

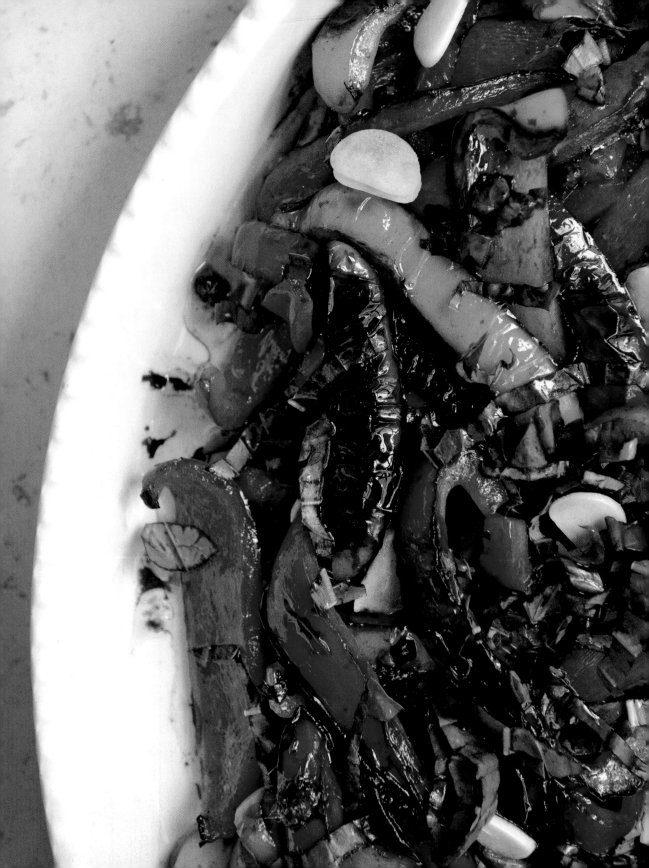

Sautéed Peppers with Capers

A chiffonade of basil is an easy way to add a bright touch of green—and the fresh taste of basil—to any dish. The process isn't complicated. Just stack, roll, and slice: after cutting off the stems, stack the leaves, roll them tightly like a cigar, and slice the roll crosswise to make slivers. As a general rule, since it's so delicate, basil should be sliced just before using and added near the very end of cooking.

You can serve this as an appetizer or side dish. My wife and I often have this with sliced bread, cheese, and a glass of wine for a snack at night. I like to include extra anchovies and lay them on top of this dish for flavor. Delicious.

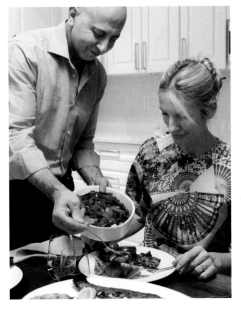

SERVES 2 TO 4

5 tablespoons extra-virgin olive oil
2 yellow bell peppers, cut
    lengthwise into ½- to 1-inch-
    wide strips
2 red bell peppers, cut lengthwise
    into ½- to 1-inch-wide strips
½ teaspoon salt
½ teaspoon black pepper
2 tablespoons balsamic vinegar
    or balsamic reduction (see
    page 77)
10 leaves fresh basil, cut into
    chiffonade (or to taste)
6 anchovies, each cut into thirds
2 tablespoons capers
2 cloves garlic, sliced

1. Put 3 tablespoons of the oil in a large pan over medium-high heat and add the bell peppers and salt. Cover and cook for 3 minutes, then uncover and stir. Cook until the peppers are fork-tender, retaining a little bit of their crunchiness, 3 to 5 minutes.

2. Add the black pepper, balsamic, basil, anchovies, and capers. Sauté for 30 seconds. The anchovies will start to melt into the mixture but will not completely dissolve. Top with the raw garlic slices and drizzle with the remaining 2 tablespoons of olive oil.

Fresh Herbs versus Dry

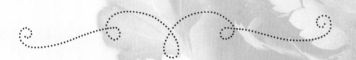

Fresh herbs are more fragrant and taste better, so it is great to use them, but in most cases, the dried versions are also good. The fresh ones are less potent so you have to use more (the ratio is about three times as much fresh herb as dry).

Herbs I always prefer fresh are: mint, basil, sage, rosemary, thyme, parsley (always flat-leaf because curly doesn't have much flavor), cilantro, and dill. I try to seek out fresh oregano too, when I can, though it's hard to find it as fragrant as I like. In general, herbs with woody stems—like oregano and bay leaves—do fine when dried, while the soft, tender herbs—like chives and parsley—do better fresh.

Dried herbs tend to work best if they're added earlier on during cooking so their flavor has time to infuse the whole dish—add them too late, and they just taste dusty. Put fresh herbs in toward the end of the cooking process so the flavor doesn't dissipate. When you add spices and herbs to cold recipes, such as dressings and dips, a brief period of refrigeration before serving will allow the flavors to blend.

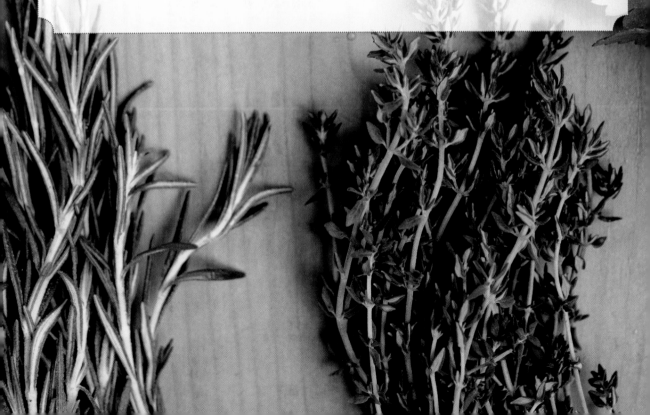

Pan-Roasted Brussels Sprouts

SERVES 6

2 pounds Brussels sprouts, trimmed and cut in half (see Note)

8 tablespoons extra-virgin olive oil

1 teaspoon salt

1 tablespoon Dijon or whole-grain mustard

1 tablespoon chopped fresh thyme

¼ cup sherry wine vinegar

1. Preheat the oven to 400°F.

2. Place the Brussels sprouts on a baking pan in a single layer. Mix them well with 2 tablespoons of the oil and ½ teaspoon of the salt and place them cut side down. Add 2 tablespoons of water to the pan and cover it with aluminum foil.

3. Bake for 10 minutes. Stir the Brussels sprouts with a spatula, and cook them for another 5 to 7 minutes uncovered.

4. Meanwhile, whisk together the mustard, remaining ½ teaspoon of salt, the thyme, and vinegar in a bowl. Slowly drizzle in the remaining 6 tablespoons of oil while whisking until they are fully incorporated.

5. While the sprouts are still hot, put them into a large bowl and toss them well with the vinaigrette.

NOTE: If you're using baby Brussels sprouts, leave them whole.

Boiled Artichokes

The artichoke is a perennial plant in the sunflower family and is believed to be a native of the Mediterranean. The "vegetable" that we eat is actually a flower bud. When shopping for fresh artichokes, look for the ones with tight leaf formation and a deep green color. They should seem heavy for their size, and the leaves should squeak when squeezed together. Avoid artichokes that look dry or have split leaves.

Interestingly, this dish is what I remember as our usual dessert in Italy. Try it after dinner with a glass of red wine.

SERVES 4

4 whole artichokes, tough outer layer removed, stems and tips trimmed
1 teaspoon salt

Juice of ½ lemon
2 cloves garlic, crushed
2 tablespoons extra-virgin olive oil

1. Layer the artichokes in a pot with enough water to cover them and add the salt, lemon juice, and garlic.
2. Bring the water to a boil over high heat, cover the pot, and simmer for 30 to 40 minutes, until the artichokes are tender. To test this, remove one artichoke from the pot and carefully pull off one of the outer leaves. It should come off easily.
3. Drain the artichokes and drizzle with the oil before serving.

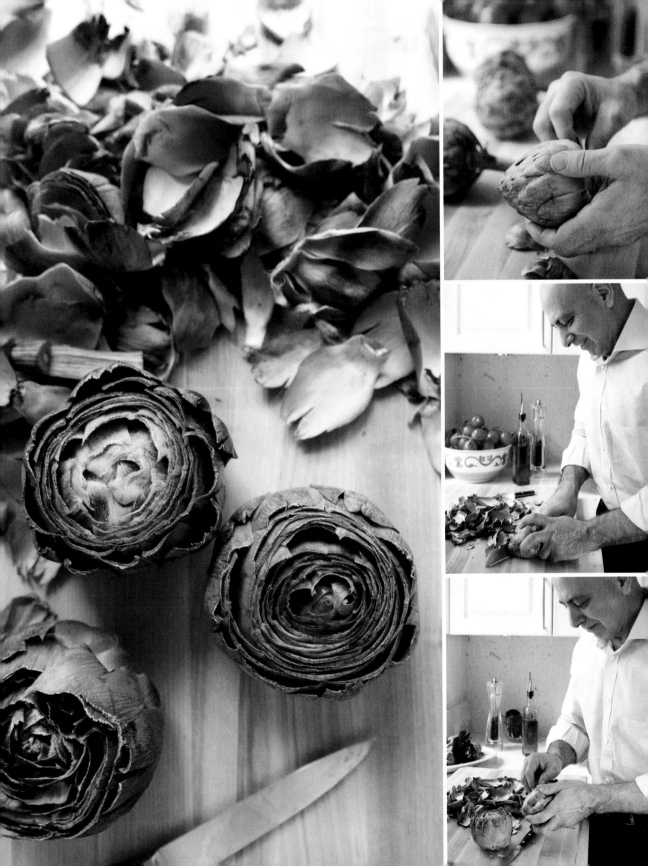

Peas with Mint

K kids

To enhance the flavor of peas, use this trick my mother taught me: add a pinch of sugar.

SERVES 4 TO 6

¼ cup extra-virgin olive oil

1 medium onion, chopped

1 pound frozen peas (2 to 3 cups), defrosted

1 teaspoon salt

1 teaspoon sugar

8 to 10 leaves fresh mint, chopped

1. Put the oil in a medium pan over medium-low heat and add the onion. Cook for 5 minutes, until it is soft.

2. Stir in the peas and ¼ cup of warm water. Add the salt, sugar, and mint and cook for 3 to 5 minutes longer.

Zucchini and Eggplant with Tomatoes

SERVES 4

1 medium eggplant, cut into
¾-inch cubes

4 tablespoons extra-virgin olive
oil

1 teaspoon salt

1 teaspoon black pepper

2 medium zucchini, cut into
¾-inch cubes

1 medium onion, sliced

¾ cup canned or fresh cherry
tomatoes (if using fresh, cut
them in half)

¼ cup white wine

3 tablespoons roughly chopped
fresh basil

1. Preheat the oven to 425°F.

2. Place the eggplant on a baking pan in a single layer. Drizzle it with half of the oil and sprinkle it with ½ teaspoon each of the salt and pepper. Mix well.

3. Bake the eggplant for 10 minutes, stirring it once or twice.

4. Put the remaining 2 tablespoons of oil in a large sauté pan over medium-high heat and add the zucchini and onion, along with the remaining ½ teaspoon each of the salt and pepper. Cook for 3 to 4 minutes.

5. Add the tomatoes, wine, and baked eggplant to the sauté pan and cook for another 4 minutes, until the zucchini is fork-tender.

6. Add the basil and serve hot.

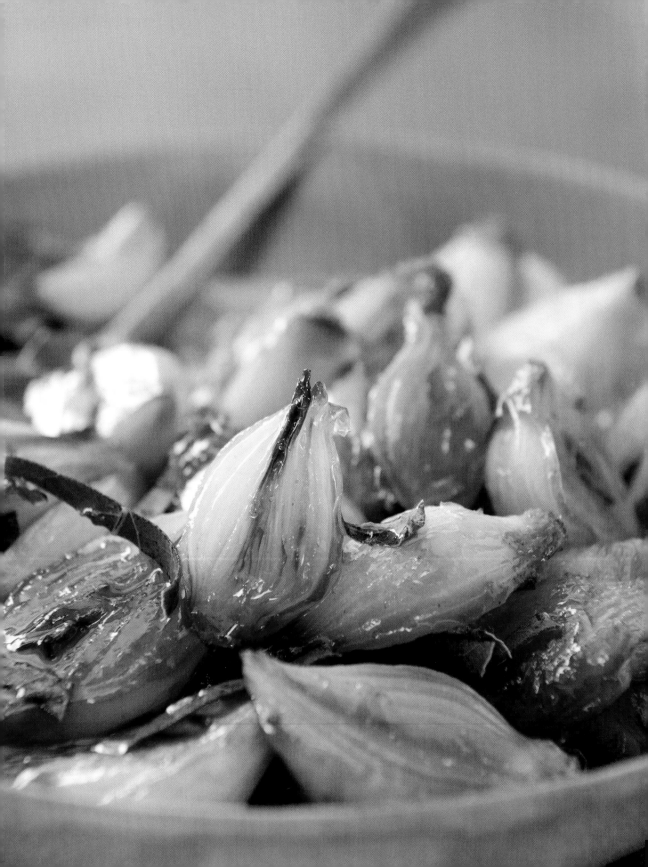

Onions Agro Dolce

Agro dolce, literally "sour and sweet," is Italy's sweet-and-sour preparation. In this recipe, the onions are caramelized. This process involves the oxidation of sugar during cooking, which browns the food and brings about a sweet, nutty flavor. This can be served as a side dish or condiment and is a wonderful accompaniment to any poultry or meat dish.

SERVES 4

1 pound baby onions
3 tablespoons extra-virgin olive
  oil
4 fresh bay leaves (see Note)

1 tablespoon brown sugar
1½ tablespoons honey
Zest of 1 lemon
6 tablespoons red wine vinegar

1. Bring a medium pot of water to a boil. Add the onions and boil them for 1 minute, then drain. Once they've cooled, peel them and cut them in half.

2. Put the oil in a large pan over high heat, and add the bay leaves and onions. Cook for 5 minutes, until the onions are slightly brown.

3. Lower the heat to medium and add the sugar, honey, and lemon zest. Cook for 3 minutes, until the onions are caramelized.

4. Add the vinegar, toss it all together, and cook for another 4 to 5 minutes. Remove and discard the bay leaves. Serve the onions hot.

NOTE: It's worth it to seek out fresh bay leaves, but you can substitute dried in a pinch.

Sautéed Broccoli Rabe

S seniors

Broccoli rabe is the Italian broccoli. Also called rapini, it's a variety of broccoli that, instead of a head, has long, thin, leafy stalks topped with tiny broccoli florets. The florets, or flowers, are quite delicate, and the leaves have a slightly bitter, pungent taste. Like its bigger cousin, broccoli rabe is one of the most nutrient-dense foods on the planet. It's packed with potassium, iron, calcium, lutein, and vitamins A, C, and K, as well as fiber.

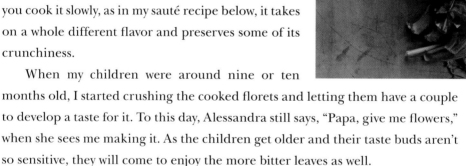

I love it and cook with it frequently. To prepare it, you need to use the tender portions, so remove the big leaves and discard them, trim the stems to about 2 inches, and discard the ends (you can save them to make broccoli rabe pesto). To simply boil broccoli rabe, place the trimmed pieces in about a quart of boiling salted water for 1 to 2 minutes. Drain it, pour about 1 tablespoon of olive oil on it, sprinkle with a pinch of salt if you like, and serve. If you cook it slowly, as in my sauté recipe below, it takes on a whole different flavor and preserves some of its crunchiness.

When my children were around nine or ten months old, I started crushing the cooked florets and letting them have a couple to develop a taste for it. To this day, Alessandra still says, "Papa, give me flowers," when she sees me making it. As the children get older and their taste buds aren't so sensitive, they will come to enjoy the more bitter leaves as well.

SERVES 2

3 tablespoons extra-virgin olive
   oil
4 cloves garlic, sliced
1 bunch broccoli rabe, washed
   and trimmed, preserving top
   3 inches of florets (see Note)
Pinch of salt

1. Put 2 tablespoons of the olive oil in a sauté pan over medium heat and add the garlic. Cook until it turns a light yellow, 1 to 2 minutes.

2. Add the trimmed broccoli rabe to the pan. If it's dry, you'll need to add about 3 tablespoons of water.

3. Allow the broccoli rabe to cook slowly over low to medium heat, while tossing every now and then. Cook it for 3 to 5 minutes, uncovered.

4. Remove the broccoli rabe from the heat, sprinkle on the salt, and drizzle the remaining 1 tablespoon of oil on top. Serve hot.

NOTE: There's no need to dry the broccoli rabe after washing it. The moisture will be needed when it's cooking.

VEGGIE-SAVING TIP: You can sauté just about any vegetable in olive oil as described here, and sprinkle with salt and pepper. Add garlic or red pepper flakes to the oil for an extra kick.

Eggplant Carpaccio

This can be an appetizer or a side dish. Serve it with a nice piece of fish or any kind of meat. Be sure to oil the grill before you cook the eggplant, because the slices are very thin and will stick otherwise.

SERVES 4

2 baby eggplants, peeled and sliced thin as a dime (see Note)

4 tablespoons extra-virgin olive oil

½ teaspoon salt

½ teaspoon black pepper

2 tablespoons finely chopped fresh mint

Juice of ½ lemon

1 small clove garlic, finely chopped

1. Heat up your grill or set a grill pan over medium-high heat. Coat the eggplant slices on both sides, using 2 tablespoons of the oil; sprinkle with the salt and pepper.

2. Grill the eggplant slices for 1 minute on each side, then set them aside to rest for 5 minutes.

3. In a small bowl, combine the remaining 2 tablespoons of oil with the mint, lemon juice, and garlic.

4. Arrange eggplant slices in a single layer on each plate and drizzle them with the dressing just before serving.

NOTE: This is best done with a mandoline.

Roasted Cauliflower

K kids **S** seniors

SERVES 6

1 head cauliflower, broken into
   1-inch florets (about 4 cups)
¼ cup extra-virgin olive oil

1 teaspoon salt
1 teaspoon black pepper
½ cup grated Fontina cheese

1. Preheat the oven to 400°F.
2. In a large bowl, mix the cauliflower florets well with the oil, salt, and pepper. Place the cauliflower on a baking pan in a single layer.
3. Roast the cauliflower for 20 minutes.
4. Sprinkle the cheese on top and roast for 5 minutes longer, then serve.

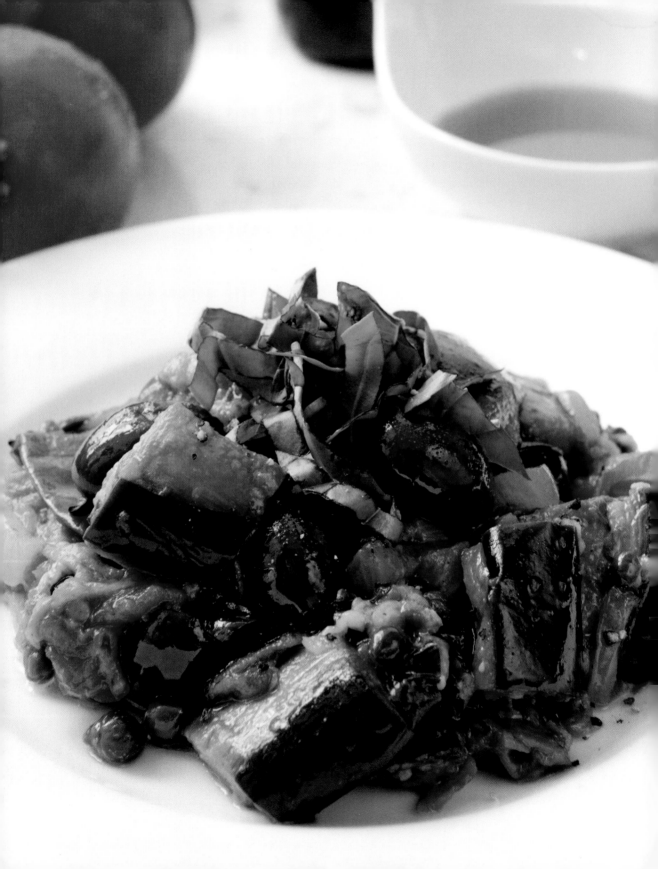

Sicilian Caponata

Caponata means cooked vegetables mixed together and usually includes eggplant. This dish has a sweet-and-sour flavor. When finished, it should be allowed to sit at room temperature for two to three hours. If you decide not to eat it until the next day, refrigerate it—the longer it sits, the better it will taste.

SERVES 6 TO 8

4 eggplants, skin removed in alternating strips (see Note) and cut into 1-inch cubes

5 plum tomatoes, cut into quarters

½ cup extra-virgin olive oil

½ tablespoon salt

1 onion, coarsely chopped

2 cloves garlic, finely chopped

½ cup Kalamata olives, pitted and halved

¼ cup capers, drained

2 tablespoons sugar

¼ cup white wine vinegar

2 tablespoons coarsely chopped fresh basil

1. Preheat the oven to broil.

2. Place the eggplants and tomatoes in one layer onto a baking pan, coat them with ¼ cup of the oil, and sprinkle them with the salt.

3. Broil them for 5 to 7 minutes until golden, tossing a couple of times.

4. Put 3 tablespoons of the olive oil in a large pan over medium heat. Add the onion and sauté for 3 to 4 minutes, until the onion pieces are soft and translucent (take care that they don't burn: stir frequently, especially around the periphery, and add a little water if needed). Add the garlic in the last minute or two.

5. Add the olives, capers, sugar, and vinegar and sauté for 3 minutes longer on medium heat.

6. Add the eggplant and tomato mixture and the remaining 1 tablespoon of oil to the pan and cook for another 2 minutes.

7. Top with the basil before serving.

NOTE: Each eggplant is partially peeled by running the peeler from top to bottom in alternating strips, with about an inch in between. The reason for this is that if you completely peel it, it'll fall apart, but if you leave all of the skin on, the skin is too tough and unpleasant to eat.

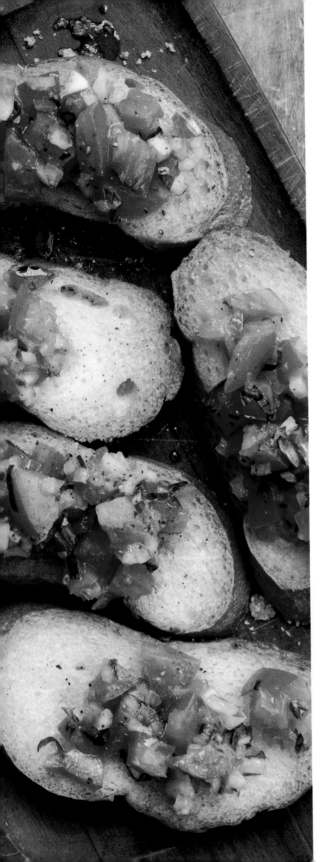

Bruschetta, Two Ways

Simple Bruschetta

Serve this vibrant, tomato-based blend on top of crusty bread, or you can use it as a tasty topping for any appetizer or entree. This one is perfect on my Baked Chicken Tenders (page 259) and Easy Baked Chicken Cutlets (page 260).

SERVES 4

¼ cup extra-virgin olive oil, plus more as needed
6 plum tomatoes, seeded and diced
3 tablespoons chopped fresh basil
½ teaspoon salt
½ teaspoon black pepper
½ medium red onion, finely chopped
½ clove garlic, finely chopped
Loaf of Italian bread

1. Preheat the oven to 450°F.
2. Combine the olive oil with the tomatoes, basil, salt, pepper, onion, and garlic in a bowl and mix well. Let the topping sit at room temperature for 30 minutes so that the flavors can blend.
3. Thinly slice the Italian bread, brush each side with olive oil, spread the slices on a baking pan, and toast them on both sides until they are golden, 4 to 5 minutes.
4. To serve, spoon some of the tomato mixture on top of each toast, drizzle with additional olive oil, and enjoy!

Ricotta and Anchovy Bruschetta

This is one of my favorite bruschetta recipes. Serve it warm for maximum flavor.

SERVES 4 TO 6

Loaf of Italian bread
5 tablespoons extra-virgin olive oil, plus more
    for serving
½ pound ricotta cheese
9 anchovy fillets, chopped
1 teaspoon freshly ground black pepper
1 teaspoon chopped thyme or rosemary

1. Preheat the oven to 450°F.

2. Thinly slice the Italian bread, brush each side with 1 tablespoon of the olive oil, spread the slices on a baking pan, and toast them until they are golden, 4 to 5 minutes.

3. While the bread is toasting, combine the rest of the ingredients in a bowl with the remaining 4 tablespoons olive oil and mix well.

4. Spread the ricotta mixture onto the toasted bread and drizzle with additional olive oil.

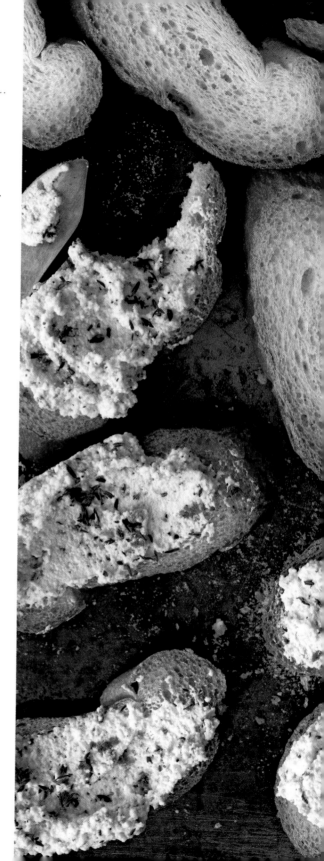

Olive Pâté

Serve this with thinly sliced toasted bread.

SERVES 4

¼ cup extra-virgin olive oil

6 anchovy fillets, chopped

Zest and juice of 1 lemon

2 cups pitted Kalamata olives

½ clove garlic, chopped

Combine all the ingredients in a food processor or blender. Blend to a finely chopped consistency. The pâté should be served at room temperature and can be stored in the refrigerator for up to 2 days.

Legumes

Ⓑ babies
Ⓚ kids
Ⓢ seniors

Bean Salad with Corn, Chickpeas, and Basil

Ⓚ kids Ⓢ seniors

Grilled fresh corn makes this recipe taste sensational, though, in a pinch, you can also use frozen or canned. The "crisp" versions of canned corn are nice, because they retain the crunchiness of fresh corn (be sure to rinse canned corn to remove excess salt). This dish is best served at room temperature.

SERVES 4 TO 6

¼ cup chopped fresh basil
3 tablespoons balsamic vinegar
1 teaspoon ground cumin
Zest and juice of 3 limes
1 teaspoon salt
1 teaspoon black pepper
⅓ cup extra-virgin olive oil
1 (14-ounce) can black beans, drained and rinsed

1 (14-ounce) can chickpeas, drained and rinsed
Kernels from 3 ears grilled corn (about 1½ cups)
3 plum tomatoes, seeded and diced

1. Combine the basil, vinegar, cumin, lime zest and juice, salt, and pepper in a small bowl. Whisk the oil in slowly.

2. In a large bowl, combine the beans, chickpeas, corn, and tomatoes. Add the dressing and toss to mix thoroughly.

Lentil Salad

In many restaurants in New York, you'll find this dish made with pancetta instead of almonds. In Sicily, my mother used almonds because they were always available and pancetta was not easy to come by, and I prefer them. They complement the other ingredients really well, give the salad a crunch, and are better for you as well.

SERVES 6

1 pound dried green or brown lentils (3 to 3½ cups cooked)

1 cup chopped celery

1 cup chopped onion

1 cup chopped carrots

2 bay leaves

¼ cup red or white wine vinegar

¼ cup white wine

¼ cup chopped fresh parsley

1 tablespoon salt

1 tablespoon black pepper

½ cup extra-virgin olive oil

½ cup sliced almonds

1. Combine the lentils, celery, onion, carrots, and bay leaves in a large pot. Add enough water to cover the vegetables by four finger-widths.

2. Bring the water to a boil, lower the heat to medium, and simmer for 20 to 30 minutes, until the lentils are tender.

3. Meanwhile, in a small bowl, combine the vinegar, wine, parsley, salt, and pepper. Whisk in the oil, adding it in a thin stream. Set the dressing aside.

4. In a sauté pan over medium heat, toast the almonds for 1 to 2 minutes. Take care that they don't burn.

5. Drain the lentils, remove the bay leaves, and return the lentils to the pot. Stir in the dressing, and cook the mixture over medium heat for 1 to 2 minutes.

6. Pour the lentil mixture into a large bowl, add the almonds (stir them in or sprinkle them on top), and serve warm or at room temperature.

Crema di Cannellini (White Bean Dip)

This is the Italian version of hummus. It is served warm, which may seem unusual—many aren't used to eating hummus warm—but it's very hearty and enjoyable. Spread it on toasted Italian bread or pita bread and drizzle olive oil over it. Refrigerate what's left and have as a snack with baby carrots or chopped vegetables.

SERVES 4

5 tablespoons extra-virgin olive oil

2 cloves garlic, chopped

2 cups dried cannellini beans, soaked overnight and cooked until tender (see page 153), or 3 (14-ounce) cans cannellini beans, drained and rinsed

1 tablespoon chopped fresh thyme

½ cup vegetable broth or water, more if needed

1 tablespoon salt

1. In a large pan, heat 2 tablespoons of the olive oil over medium-high heat. Add the garlic and cook until it turns a light yellow.

2. Add the beans, thyme, vegetable broth, and salt, and cook for approximately 3 minutes.

3. Place the contents of the pan into a blender and puree until it is smooth. You may add a bit more liquid if the consistency is too thick.

4. Place the puree in a serving bowl and drizzle the remaining 3 tablespoons of oil over the top to serve.

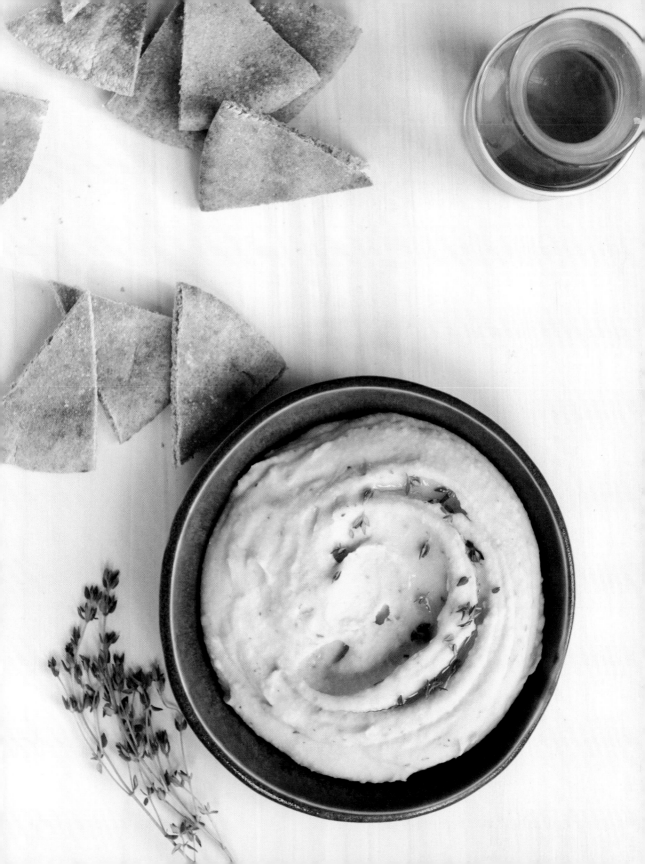

Simple Bean Salad

⑤ seniors

SERVES 4

1 (14-ounce) can chickpeas, drained and rinsed

1 (14-ounce) can cannellini beans, drained and rinsed

1 tablespoon chopped fresh basil

1 teaspoon chopped fresh thyme

½ teaspoon salt

½ teaspoon black pepper

½ medium onion, chopped

3 tablespoons extra-virgin olive oil

2 stalks celery, chopped

4 radishes, sliced

Juice of ½ lemon

1 tablespoon red wine vinegar

This preparation couldn't be simpler: mix everything together in a large bowl.

Swiss Chard and Cannellini Beans alla Alessandra

K kids **S** seniors

This delicious side dish was my daughter Alessandra's idea. We were preparing a similar dish with pasta, and she sampled it before it was ready and said, "Papa, I like this without the pasta!" And so a new vegetable side dish was born in the Acquista household.

SERVES 4 TO 6

2 bunches Swiss chard

1 teaspoon salt

7 tablespoons extra-virgin olive oil

4 cloves garlic, sliced

3 (14-ounce) cans cannellini beans, drained and rinsed (4 to 5 cups)

Black pepper, optional

1. Place a large pot of water on the stove to boil.

2. Meanwhile, prepare the Swiss chard: separate the leaves from the stems and chop the leaves into 2- to 3-inch pieces. Cut the stems into 1-inch-long strips about ¼ inch wide.

3. Add the salt and chard stems to the boiling water and cook them for 5 minutes.

4. Add the chard leaves to the pot and cook for another 2 minutes. Reserve ½ cup of the cooking water, then drain the Swiss chard well.

5. Put 3 tablespoons of the olive oil in a skillet over medium heat and add the garlic.

6. When the garlic turns yellow, add the chard leaves and stems. Cook it on high heat for 1 minute and then add the cannellini beans. Stir the Swiss chard and beans together and sauté them for 1 to 2 minutes more. Add a few tablespoons of the reserved water to the mixture to give it a loose consistency.

7. Add pepper to taste.

8. Drizzle the remaining 4 tablespoons of olive oil over the dish and serve.

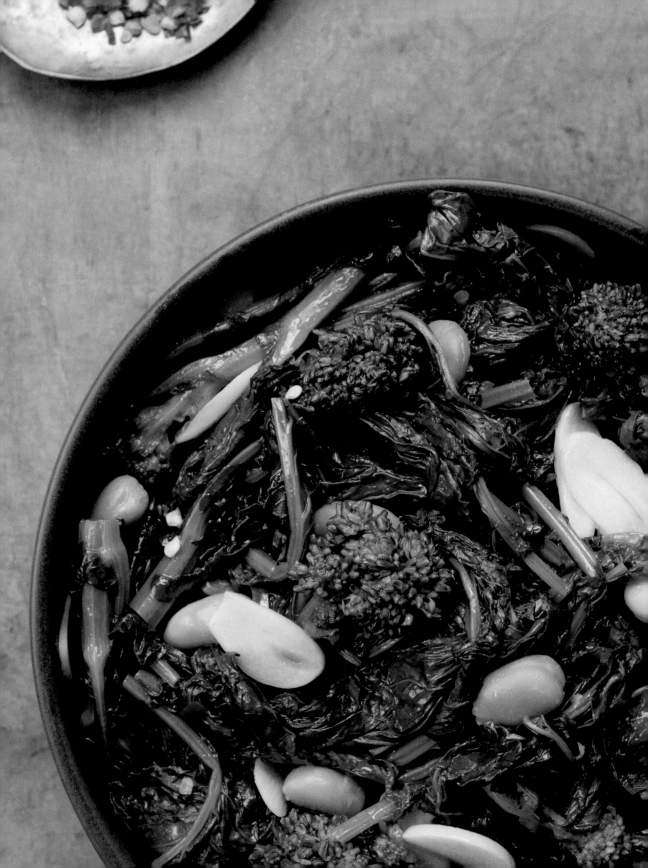

Fava Beans with Broccoli Rabe

⑤ seniors

SERVES 4

1 (28-ounce) package frozen
   fava beans (4 to 5 cups)
7 cloves garlic, 4 crushed and
   3 sliced
1½ teaspoons salt
¼ cup extra-virgin olive oil

2 bunches broccoli rabe, washed
   and trimmed, keeping only
   the top 2 to 3 inches of the
   florets and stems to cook
½ teaspoon red pepper flakes

1. Wash the frozen fava beans under cold water for 1 minute.

2. Place the fava beans in a pot with just enough cold water to cover them (if you put them in hot water, the skins will stay hard).

3. Add the crushed garlic to the pot. Bring the mixture to a boil over high heat, then lower the heat and simmer, covered, for 15 to 20 minutes.

4. Add 1 teaspoon of the salt 1 to 2 minutes before the end of the cooking time.

5. Meanwhile, put 2 tablespoons of the olive oil in a pan over medium-high heat and sauté the sliced garlic for 1 minute, until it is golden yellow.

6. Add the broccoli rabe, the remaining ½ teaspoon of salt, the red pepper flakes, and 2 tablespoons of water to the pan, and lower the heat to medium. Cook the broccoli rabe slowly for 2 to 4 minutes, tossing it and adding a little bit more water if the pan gets too dry.

7. Drain the fava beans and add them to the broccoli rabe; cook for 30 seconds longer.

8. Place the vegetables into a large serving bowl, and drizzle the remaining 2 tablespoons of olive oil over the top.

Pasta and Other Grains

B babies
K kids
S seniors

Cavatelli with Roman Cauliflower

Roman cauliflower (also known as Romanesco) grows as a peculiar spiky, conical head, and instead of florets as in regular cauliflower, it projects cones with tiny cones upon cones—a kind of fractal of nature's making. It comes in various hues of white, purple, and green and has a nutty, more intense flavor compared with regular cauliflower. Unfortunately it's not always easy to find in many stores in the US, though sources like farmers' markets often carry it, as do Italian specialty shops. You can substitute standard cauliflower for this if you can't find the Roman variety. It breaks into florets and cooks the same way.

SERVES 6

2 tablespoons salt

1 medium head cauliflower, cut into 1-inch florets (about 4 cups)

6 tablespoons extra-virgin olive oil, plus extra for drizzling

3 shallots, finely chopped

1 teaspoon red pepper flakes

3 anchovy fillets, chopped

1 pound cavatelli

¼ cup grated pecorino cheese, plus more for serving

1. Add ½ tablespoon of the salt and the cauliflower to a large pot of water and bring to a boil over high heat.

2. Cook for 3 minutes, then remove the cauliflower from the water. Retain the water.

3. Put half of the cauliflower into a blender along with 1 cup of the cooking water and 2 tablespoons of the oil. Blend until it turns into a puree. This will be the sauce for your pasta. You may need to add more of the cooking water to reach the desired consistency (as loose as tomato puree).

4. Heat the remaining 4 tablespoons of oil in a pan over medium heat. Add the shallots, red pepper flakes, and anchovies. Sauté for 1 minute.

5. Increase the heat to high and add the reserved cauliflower florets. Sauté for 2 minutes while stirring.

6. Add the puree to the pan and sauté for 30 to 40 seconds while stirring.

continued >

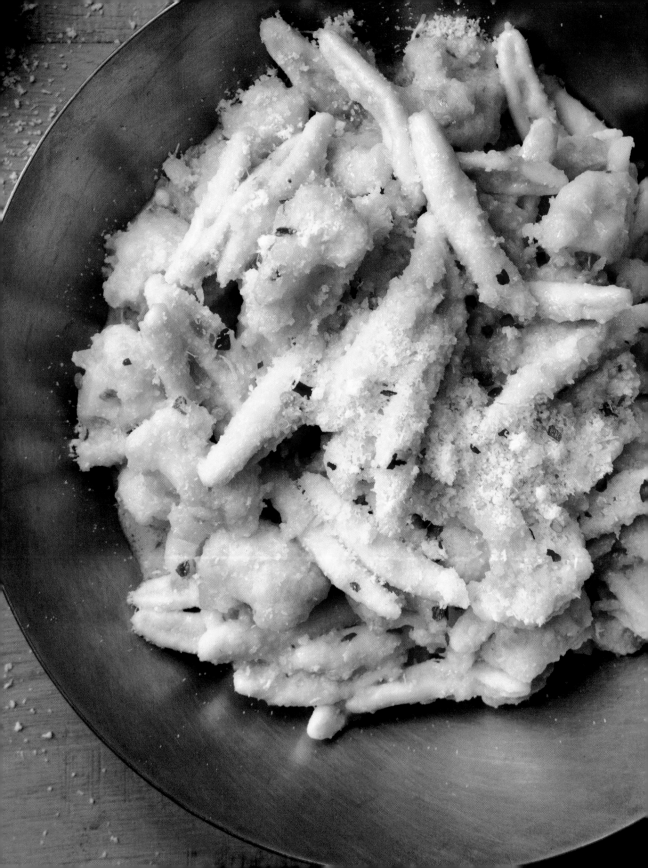

7. To the pot with the reserved cauliflower cooking water, add the remaining 1½ tablespoons of salt, return the water to a boil over high heat, and add the cavatelli. Cook according to the package instructions until al dente, 5 to 8 minutes.

8. Reserve ½ cup of the pasta cooking water. Drain the pasta, stir it into the pan with the sauce, and cook everything together for 30 seconds. Add a couple more tablespoons of the pasta cooking water for a looser consistency, if desired.

9. Remove the pan from the heat and stir in the cheese.

10. Drizzle each serving with olive oil and serve with extra grated cheese for sprinkling.

Rigatoni with Broiled Eggplant, Swordfish, and Mint

....

This is a recipe I ordered in Puglia, Italy. As I was eating it, my children loved it so much they requested an order as well, which I then split between the three of them. The chef graciously gave me the recipe. Serve this with grated Parmigiano or pecorino cheese for the table.

SERVES 6 TO 8

1 large eggplant, skin removed in alternating strips about 1 inch wide, cut into 1-inch cubes

9 tablespoons extra-virgin olive oil

1 tablespoon plus 1½ teaspoons salt

1 large onion, chopped

3 anchovy fillets in oil, chopped

½ teaspoon red pepper flakes

1 pound swordfish, cut into ½-inch cubes

Splash of white wine

1 pound rigatoni pasta

¼ cup chopped fresh mint

1. Set the oven to broil. In a bowl, mix the eggplant with 2 tablespoons of the oil and ½ teaspoon of the salt. Spread it in a single layer on a baking pan.

2. Broil the eggplant until golden, stirring to prevent burning, about 5 minutes.

3. In a large sauté pan, heat 2 tablespoons of the oil over medium heat; add the onion, anchovies, and red pepper flakes, and cook until the onion is softened, about 5 minutes.

4. Increase the heat to high, add 2 more tablespoons of oil, the swordfish, and 1 teaspoon of the salt, and sauté for 30 seconds; add the wine.

5. Cook for 1 minute, add the eggplant, cook for 30 seconds, then remove the pan from the heat.

6. Bring a large pot of water to a boil over high heat. Add the remaining 1 tablespoon of salt and the rigatoni. Cook the pasta according to the package instructions until al dente. Drain well.

7. Add the rigatoni to the pan with the swordfish and eggplant mixture. Add the mint and the remaining 3 tablespoons of oil, stir well, and serve.

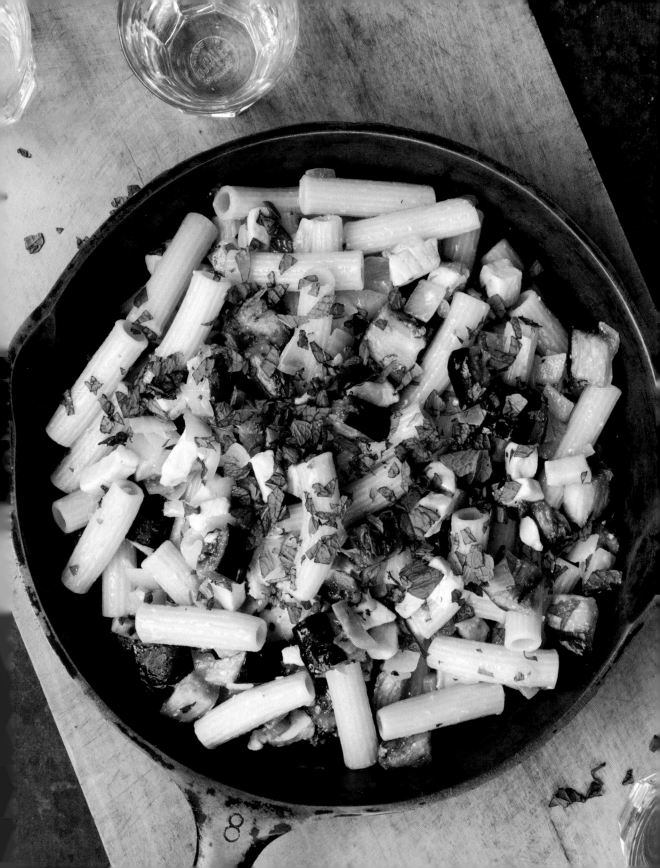

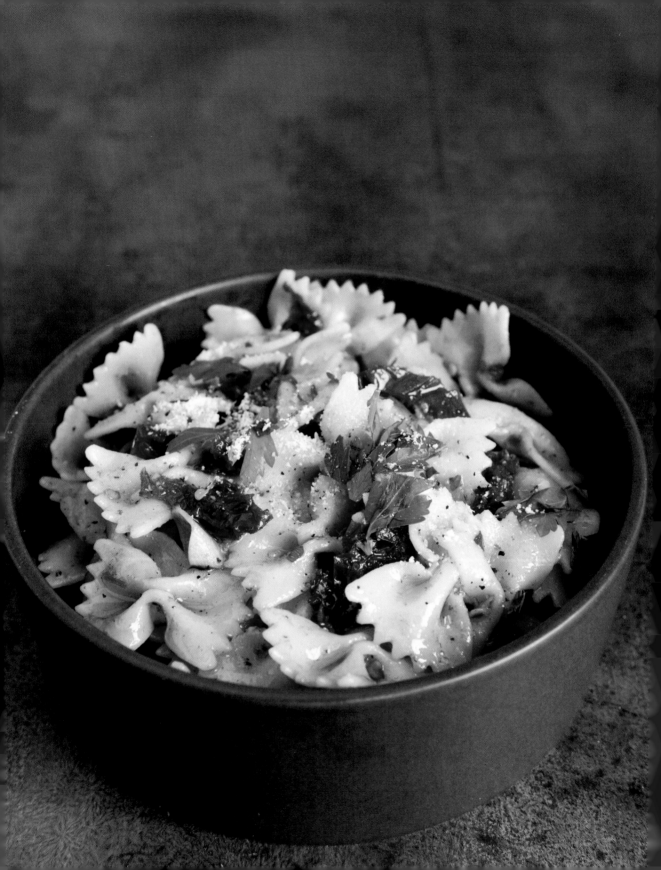

Farfalle Pasta with Pecorino Cheese and Sun-Dried Tomatoes

Sun-dried tomatoes and pecorino cheese are both very common in Sicily. Sun-dried tomatoes are easily made because the sun is so hot and drying—it only takes two to three days of sitting in the sun to desiccate them. Once dried, they can last for a year or two in a plastic bag, which is what my mother used to do. When you were ready to eat them, you'd put them in oil for a day or so to soften them up, adding salt, oregano, and garlic as a flavorful marinade. Or people jarred them in oil once they were dried as another way to preserve them.

SERVES 6

4 tablespoons extra-virgin
  olive oil
½ teaspoon red pepper flakes
5 cloves garlic, sliced
5 anchovy fillets, chopped
¼ cup white wine
⅔ cup sun-dried tomatoes in
  olive oil, sliced

1 tablespoon salt
1 pound farfalle pasta
1 teaspoon black pepper
¼ cup grated pecorino cheese
2 tablespoons chopped fresh
  parsley

1. In a heated pan, add 2 tablespoons of the oil, the red pepper flakes, garlic, and anchovies. With the back of a wooden spoon, mash the anchovies into the oil until they melt. Add the wine and cook for 30 seconds, then add the sun-dried tomatoes. Cook for additional 30 seconds.

2. Bring a large pot of water to a boil over high heat. Add the salt and the farfalle and cook according to the package instructions until al dente. When the pasta is done, reserve ½ cup of the pasta cooking water before draining it. Stir the drained pasta into the pan with the anchovy mixture, along with the reserved pasta water.

3. Remove the pan from the heat and stir in the black pepper, pecorino cheese, and parsley.

4. Drizzle the pasta with the remaining 2 tablespoons of olive oil.

Fusilli with Broccoli Rabe and Radicchio

S seniors

SERVES 6

2 bunches broccoli rabe

8 tablespoons extra-virgin olive oil

12 large cloves garlic (the more, the better!), sliced

½ teaspoon red pepper flakes

4 anchovy fillets, chopped, optional

2 medium heads radicchio, roughly sliced into 2-inch pieces

1½ tablespoons salt

1 pound fusilli or any short pasta

½ cup grated pecorino or Parmigiano cheese

1. Wash and trim the broccoli rabe, cutting no more than 2 to 3 inches from the florets. Chop the remainder of the stems into ¼-inch pieces. Set aside.

2. Use 2 tablespoons of the oil to coat the bottom of a large pan over medium heat and add the garlic, red pepper flakes, and anchovies, if desired. Sauté until the garlic is golden brown and the anchovies have melted into the oil.

3. Increase the heat to medium-high and add the radicchio. Sauté for 1 to 2 minutes, then add the broccoli rabe and ½ tablespoon of the salt.

4. Lower the heat to medium and let the mixture cook for 3 minutes, stirring occasionally. You want the broccoli rabe to retain a little crunchiness.

5. Bring a large pot of water to a boil over high heat. Add the remaining 1 tablespoon of salt and the fusilli and cook according to the package instructions until al dente. When it is done, reserve ¼ cup of the cooking water and drain the pasta.

6. Add the pasta and reserved pasta water to the pan with the broccoli rabe; cook for another 30 seconds to 1 minute.

7. Turn off the heat, add the remaining 6 tablespoons of oil, and stir in a good amount of the grated cheese. Top the individual portions with a sprinkling of the remaining cheese, and serve.

> **VEGGIE-SAVING TIP:** Add a mix of leftover veggies to any semolina pasta with some olive oil, a little grated Parmigiano cheese, salt, and pepper. The added complex carbohydrates and fiber of the vegetables slow digestion, so the meal lowers your blood sugar less than it would otherwise.

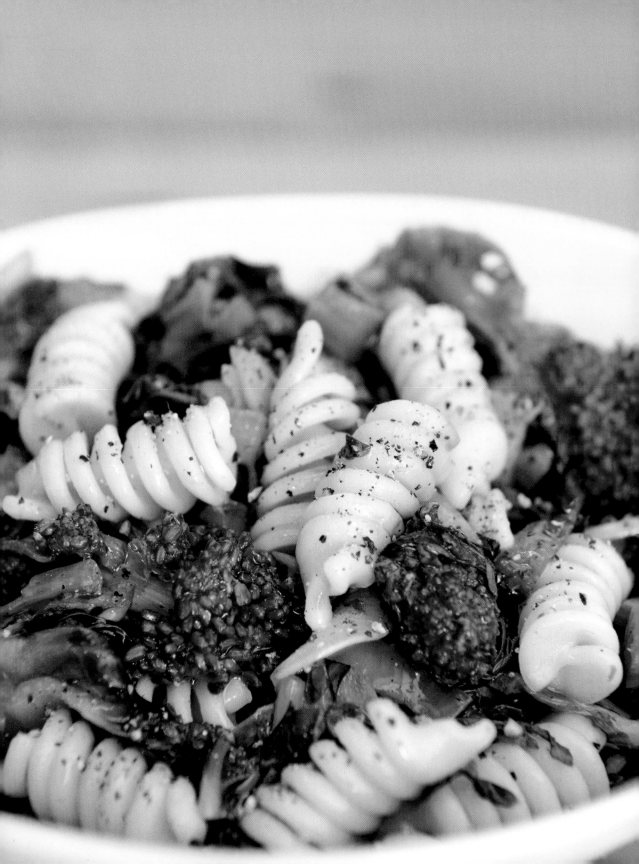

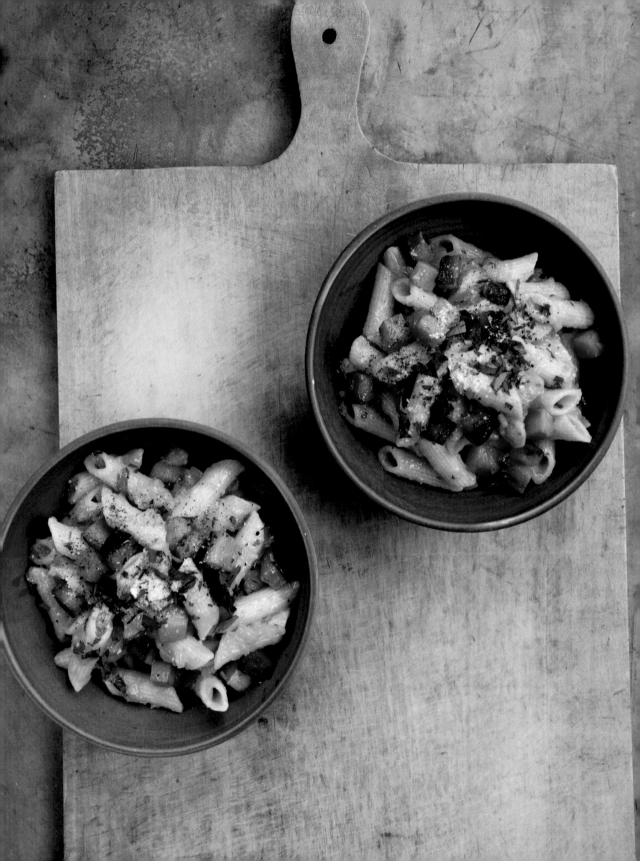

Penne with Roasted Butternut Squash

B babies K kids S seniors

SERVES 6

1 pound butternut squash,
    peeled and cut into ¼-inch
    cubes
6 tablespoons extra-virgin olive
    oil
1 tablespoon plus 1 teaspoon
    salt, optional

1 pound penne pasta
1 large onion, finely chopped
4 tablespoons grated Parmigiano
    cheese
2 tablespoons chopped fresh
    parsley
1 teaspoon black pepper

1. Preheat the oven to 425°F.

2. Toss the squash cubes in a bowl with 1 tablespoon of the oil and ½ teaspoon of the salt (if using) and mix well. Spread onto a baking pan in a single layer and roast for 20 to 30 minutes until soft. Increase the oven temperature to broil and broil the squash for 2 minutes more.

3. When the squash is almost done, bring a large pot of water to a boil over high heat. Add 1 tablespoon of the salt (if using) and the penne and cook according to the package instructions until al dente. Reserve ⅓ cup of the cooking water and drain the pasta.

4. Place half of the squash into a blender along with the reserved pasta water and puree until it is smooth. It should have the consistency of tomato sauce.

5. Put 2 tablespoons of the oil in a large pan over low heat. Add the onion and the remaining ½ teaspoon of salt (if using) and cook until the onion is softened.

6. Add the squash puree and roasted squash cubes to the onion, and sauté for 1 minute.

7. Stir in the drained pasta, and remove the pan from the heat.

8. Stir in the Parmigiano, parsley, and pepper, and drizzle with the remaining 3 tablespoons of oil.

Orecchiette with Zucchini and Ricotta Salata

K kids

Ricotta salata is the pressed, dried, and aged version of the creamy cheese you're used to buying in the refrigerated section of the market. If you cannot find ricotta salata, use pecorino instead.

SERVES 6

½ cup extra-virgin olive oil

3 medium zucchini, cut into
½-inch cubes

1 tablespoon plus 1 teaspoon
salt

6 tablespoons chopped fresh
mint

1 cup grated ricotta salata or
pecorino

1 pound orecchiette pasta

½ teaspoon black pepper

1. Heat ¼ cup of the olive oil in a pan over medium to high heat, and add the zucchini, ½ teaspoon of the salt, and 1 tablespoon of the mint. Sauté, stirring, until the zucchini cubes are golden. Add ½ teaspoon of the salt.

2. In a large serving bowl, mix the ricotta salata or pecorino cheese, 4 tablespoons of the mint, and the remaining ¼ cup of olive oil.

3. Bring a large pot of water to a boil over high heat. Add the remaining 1 tablespoon of salt and the orecchiette and cook according to the package instructions until al dente. When it is done, reserve ¼ cup of the cooking water and drain the pasta. Add the reserved pasta water to the cheese mixture.

4. Add the drained pasta to the bowl with the cheese mixture and toss.

5. Add the zucchini and the pepper and toss. Top with the remaining 1 tablespoon of mint.

> TIP: You can swap out some of the zucchini in this dish for yellow squash for a more colorful presentation.

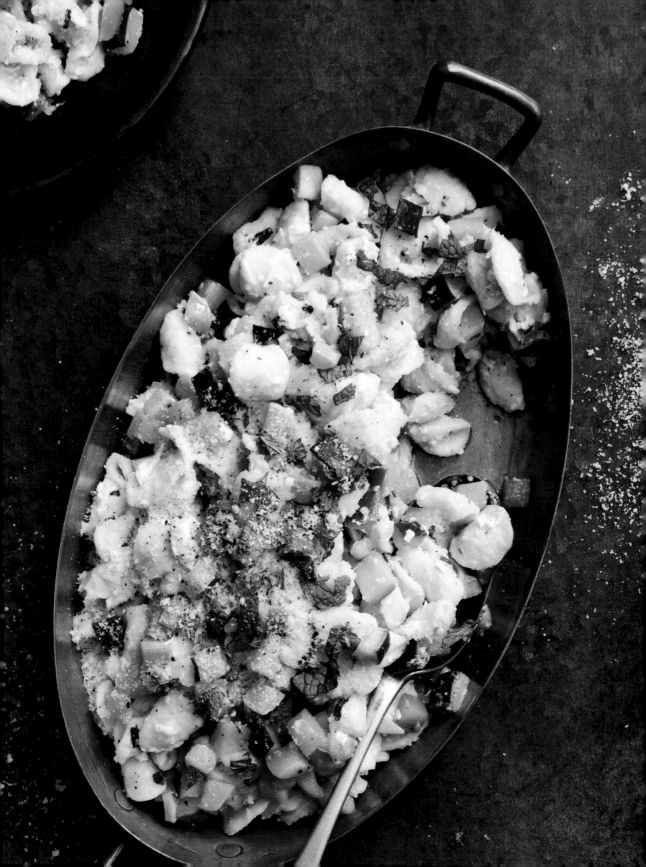

Short Pasta with Tuna, Cherry Tomatoes, and Shrimp

An alternative to preparing this dish with fresh cherry tomatoes is to use ¼ cup of sun-dried tomatoes.

SERVES 6

- 6 tablespoons extra-virgin olive oil
- 1 teaspoon red pepper flakes
- 1 medium onion, chopped
- 1 (6-ounce) can tuna in oil, drained
- ½ pound baby shrimp or rock shrimp
- 1 tablespoon plus 1 teaspoon salt
- ¼ cup white wine
- 1 tablespoon fennel seeds
- ¾ cup cherry or grape tomatoes, cut in half
- 1 pound short pasta, such as penne, rigatoni, or fusilli

1. Put 3 tablespoons of the oil in a large pan over low heat. Add the pepper flakes and onion and cook until the onion pieces are soft.

2. Increase the heat to high, add the tuna, shrimp, and 1 teaspoon of the salt and cook for 1 minute while stirring.

3. Add the wine, bring it to a boil, and cook for 1 minute.

4. Add the fennel seeds and tomatoes and cook for 1 minute.

5. Bring a large pot of water to a boil over high heat. Add the remaining 1 tablespoon of salt and the pasta and cook according to the package instructions until al dente. Reserve ½ cup of the cooking water and drain the pasta.

6. Stir the drained pasta and reserved cooking water into the pan with the tuna mixture. Cook for 30 seconds, drizzle with the remaining 3 tablespoons of olive oil, and serve.

Pasta with Fava Beans and Radicchio

....

S seniors

I keep frozen fava beans on hand for a quick legume-rich meal with pasta. If you cannot find frozen fava beans, you can use canned. You can also use fresh fava beans, though they require a lot of work to prepare.

SERVES 6

1 pound fava beans (frozen and thawed, canned, or fresh)

1 tablespoon plus ½ teaspoon salt

6 tablespoons extra-virgin olive oil

1 medium onion, chopped

3 cloves garlic, crushed

1 teaspoon red pepper flakes

6 anchovies in oil, chopped

2 medium heads radicchio, roughly sliced

1 pound short pasta such as penne, rigatoni, ziti, or fusilli

½ cup grated pecorino cheese

1. If using thawed or fresh fava beans, place them in a pan with enough cold water to cover. Bring to a boil, then cook for 15 to 20 minutes, until tender. One minute before draining the water, add ½ teaspoon of the salt. Drain the fava beans.

2. Heat 2 tablespoons of the oil in a large pan over low heat; add the onion, garlic, pepper flakes, and anchovies. Cook until the onion pieces are soft, about 5 minutes.

3. Raise the heat and add the radicchio. Sauté while stirring for 1 to 2 minutes. Add the fava beans (whether thawed, fresh, or canned) and cook for another 2 minutes.

4. Bring a large pot of water to a boil over high heat. Add the remaining 1 tablespoon of salt and the pasta and cook according to the package instructions until al dente. When it is done, reserve ½ cup of the cooking water and drain the pasta.

5. Add the reserved pasta cooking water to the pan, followed by the drained pasta, and cook for another 30 seconds.

6. Remove the pan from the heat, stir in the cheese, and drizzle with the remaining 4 tablespoons of oil.

Tagliatelle Aeolian-Style

....

This recipe is from the Aeolian Islands, a group of seven small islands off the coast of Sicily. They are volcanic in origin (two of them are still active), set amid turquoise waters and dramatic scenery. Capers are very common there and grow wild as well as being cultivated. The favorite dishes of the islands feature seafood and capers.

SERVES 4

2 large ripe, beefsteak tomatoes, or 4 plum tomatoes

1 eggplant, peeled in alternating strips and cut into ¾-inch cubes

⅓ cup extra-virgin olive oil

1 tablespoon plus ¾ teaspoon salt

2 cloves garlic, crushed

2 tablespoons capers, drained

1 teaspoon dried oregano

½ cup white wine

1 handful pine nuts

½ teaspoon red pepper flakes

½ pound fresh tagliatelle, or ¾ pound spaghetti

¾ pound fresh tuna, cut into ½-inch cubes

1. Prepare the oven to broil.

2. Bring a pot of water to a boil over high heat. Score the bottom of the tomatoes and poach them in the water for 1 minute, then remove and discard the skins and cut the tomatoes into ½-inch pieces, reserving the juice as well.

3. Place the eggplant on a baking sheet and toss it with 3 tablespoons of the oil and ¼ teaspoon of the salt. Broil it for 5 to 7 minutes, stirring every couple of minutes. Remove the eggplant from the oven when it turns golden yellow and set it aside.

4. To a pan over medium heat, add the remainder of the oil and the garlic and sauté until it turns golden.

5. Add the tomatoes with their juice, capers, oregano, wine, pine nuts, red pepper flakes, and ¼ teaspoon of the salt and let the mixture cook over medium heat for 3 to 4 minutes.

6. Meanwhile, add 1 tablespoon of the salt to a large pot of water and bring it to a boil. Add the pasta and cook until it is al dente, 3 to 4 minutes. If using dried

spaghetti, cook it for 8 to 10 minutes. Reserve ¼ cup of the cooking water and drain the pasta.

7. When the tomato sauce has cooked for about 3 minutes, sprinkle the remaining ¼ teaspoon of salt over the pieces of tuna and add them to the pan; cook for another minute.

8. Add the diced eggplant (along with its olive oil) to the pot with the sauce and stir.

9. Immediately add the drained pasta and the reserved cooking water to the sauce and warm them together for just 30 seconds, so as not to overcook the tuna. Serve hot.

Pasta Is to Be Enjoyed, Not Feared

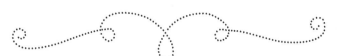

In the 1950s and '60s, pasta was a big part of the Sicilian diet, since it was high in fiber and kept you full when no one could afford meat or any kind of animal fat.

People would mill their own flour. They would bring their wheat to a mill and then take the flour home and use it to make bread and pasta. The wheat was not highly processed and refined—it was just ground—so it was healthy.

I eat pasta at least once a day, sometimes twice! Don't be afraid of carbs. If you're watching your weight, be sure to get pasta like durum semolina or whole wheat pasta that is not highly refined, and don't overcook it—this will keep it lower on the glycemic index scale. By combining lesser-refined al dente pasta with a wholesome sauce such as a tomato base, vegetable mix, and/or seafood, you will have prepared a very filling, nutritious, well-balanced meal for the dieter and nondieter alike.

Linguine with Swordfish and Almonds

SERVES 4

⅓ cup raw almonds

6 tablespoons extra-virgin olive oil

1 clove garlic

10 cherry tomatoes, cut into small pieces

2 tablespoons tomato sauce

2 tablespoons chopped fresh parsley, plus more for garnish

¼ cup white wine

½ teaspoon red pepper flakes

⅔ pound swordfish, cut into ½-inch cubes

1 tablespoon salt

¾ pound linguine

1. In a small dry pan, toast the almonds over low heat, then chop them and set aside.

2. Heat 2 tablespoons of the olive oil in a saucepan over medium heat. Add the garlic and cook until it is lightly browned, then add the tomatoes, tomato sauce, parsley, white wine, and red pepper flakes.

3. Let the mixture cook for about 5 minutes, then add the fish cubes and cook for 1 to 2 minutes longer.

4. Bring a large pot of water to a boil over high heat. Add the salt and the linguine and cook according to the package instructions until al dente. When the pasta is done, reserve ½ cup of the cooking water and drain the pasta.

5. Add the drained pasta to the sauce and sauté over medium heat for about 30 seconds, mixing well. If it's too dry, add a few tablespoons of the reserved pasta water.

6. Transfer the pasta to a serving dish, drizzle it with the remaining 4 tablespoons of olive oil, and garnish it with the chopped almonds and additional chopped parsley.

Ditalini Pasta with Ricotta

B babies **K** kids

This is a great, easy recipe that kids will love. You can use any short pasta for this dish; I like ditalini, which is like short penne. Be aware that ricotta will break down if it gets cooked, so make sure the pan is off the heat before you add it—though the ingredients should be stirred in while the pasta is really hot.

SERVES 3 CHILDREN

½ tablespoon salt, optional

⅓ pound ditalini or any short pasta

½ pound ricotta, preferably fresh

2 tablespoons extra-virgin olive oil

2 tablespoons grated Parmigiano cheese

1. Bring a medium pot of water to a boil over high heat. Add the salt (if using) and the pasta; cook until tender, 8 to 10 minutes. Reserve 2 to 3 tablespoons of the pasta water.

2. Drain the pasta, return it to the pan, and while it is still hot, add the ricotta, olive oil, and cheese. Stir to combine. If a less dense consistency is desired, stir in reserved pasta water to achieve the desired thickness.

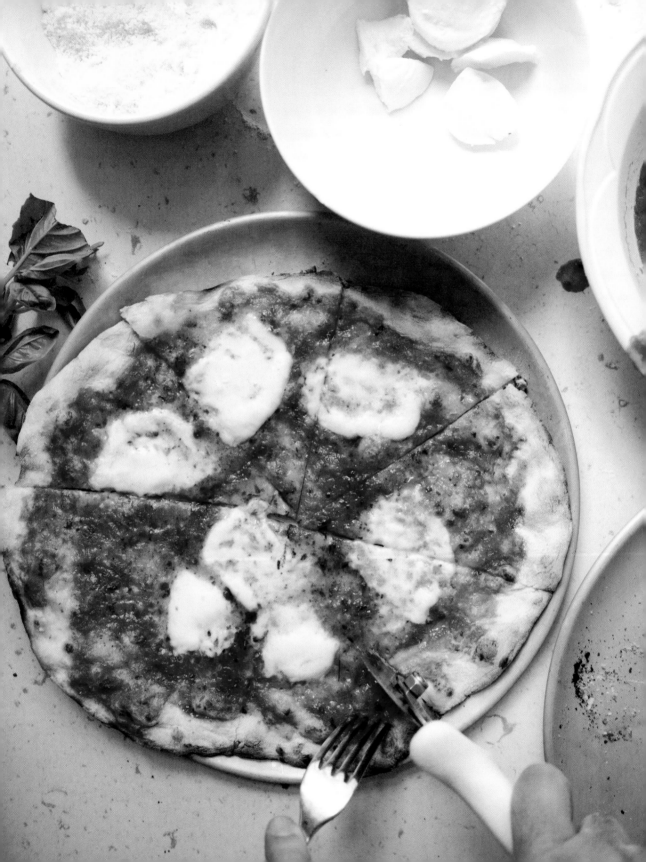

Easy Pizza

K kids

If you wish to lure your bambini into the kitchen, there's no better way than making pizza together. Children like to work with dough and love to help with that. When we make pizza, my little ones help chop whatever I'm making. Alessandra will put her hand on mine while I protect her from the blade, and she giggles and chatters to me while we do it. Even my younger ones, Nicholas and Sal, can join in the simplicity of spreading fresh tomato sauce and sprinkling cheese I have grated for them. While pizza is generally not a dish you have to woo your children to eat, the concept of inviting them into the process of food preparation inspires their interest as well as their taste buds in the meal you have prepared together. Plus, at home you can make a much healthier version than the ones in stores and restaurants—and it is just as tasty.

I buy my dough premade, because I don't care to spend the time to make it myself. I get it from our local pizzeria, but you can also find it at the supermarket. Leave it at room temperature for 30 minutes before using it.

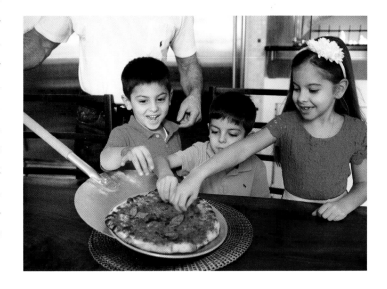

TIP: Give your children jobs to help you when making pizza. In my home, one child will get a pinch of salt and gets to sprinkle the salt on, while one will be in charge of sprinkling the pepper. Someone will get the job of sprinkling the oregano, which disperses better if it's sprinkled from high up, so they have fun with that. They love that everyone has a responsibility, and it draws them into the kitchen.

continued >

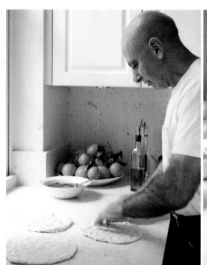
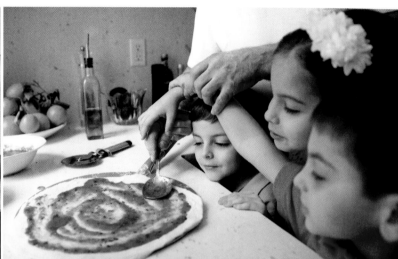
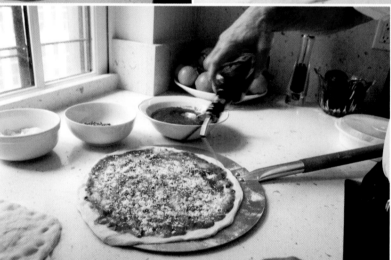
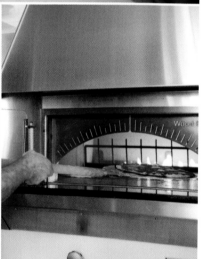
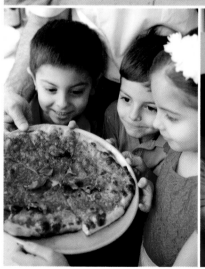
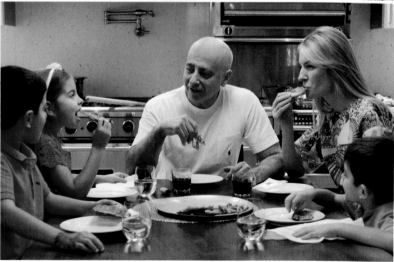

2½ tablespoons extra-virgin olive
   oil

1 pound pizza dough

1 (14-ounce) can crushed
   tomatoes, or 1½ cups crushed
   fresh tomatoes

1 tablespoon chopped fresh
   basil

¼ cup grated Parmigiano or
   pecorino cheese

6 ounces fresh mozzarella, cut
   into 1-inch cubes

1 teaspoon salt

1 teaspoon black pepper

¾ teaspoon dried oregano

1. Preheat the oven to 375°F and set the oven rack at the lowest position.

2. Using your hands, coat a nonstick pizza pan with ½ tablespoon of the oil (kids enjoy doing this).

3. Stretch the dough onto the pizza pan, and cut any excess dough away from the lip of the pan.

4. Spread the tomatoes evenly onto the dough and sprinkle them with basil, cheeses, salt, pepper, and oregano.

5. Drizzle the remaining 2 tablespoons of oil over the pizza and bake it for 20 to 30 minutes. Check the bottom of the pizza occasionally; when it has turned slightly brown, the pizza is ready.

Orecchiette with Bread Crumbs and Broccoli Rabe

Ⓢ seniors

SERVES 6

½ loaf stale Italian bread, cut into 1-inch cubes

7 tablespoons extra-virgin olive oil

6 cloves garlic, 5 sliced and 1 minced

3 anchovy fillets, chopped

1 tablespoon plus ½ teaspoon salt

2 bunches broccoli rabe, washed and trimmed

1 teaspoon red pepper flakes

1 pound orecchiette pasta

½ teaspoon black pepper

¼ cup grated Parmigiano or pecorino cheese

1. Preheat the oven to 425°F.

2. Spread the cut bread pieces on a baking pan in a single layer and sprinkle them with 1 tablespoon of the oil. Mix well and bake for 10 to 15 minutes, stirring a couple of times, until the bread is golden.

3. Put the toasted bread into a blender with the minced garlic and the anchovies. Blend until the mixture turns into bread crumbs.

4. Add 1 tablespoon of the salt to a large pot of water and bring it to a boil over high heat.

5. Cut the broccoli rabe into 2- to 3-inch florets, then cut the stems into ½-inch pieces. Blanch the broccoli rabe stems for 1 minute in the boiling water. Strain out the stems and set aside. Keep the water at a boil.

6. Place 3 tablespoons of the oil in a large pan over medium heat; add the sliced garlic and the red pepper flakes. Cook until the garlic is golden.

7. Add the broccoli rabe florets and stems, stirring well. Cook for 2 to 3 minutes. Add the remaining ½ teaspoon of salt. Lower the heat to medium, cover the pan, and cook for 30 seconds.

8. Add the orecchiette to the same pot of boiling water and cook according to the

package instructions until al dente. When it is done, reserve ¼ cup of the cooking water and drain the pasta.

9. Add the drained orecchiette to the broccoli rabe, along with the reserved cooking water. Cook for another 30 seconds.

10. Sprinkle with the remaining 3 tablespoons of oil while stirring, and add the black pepper.

11. Remove the pan from the heat and stir in the grated cheese. Sprinkle each portion of pasta generously with the bread crumbs and serve.

Anchovies

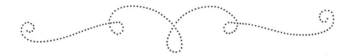

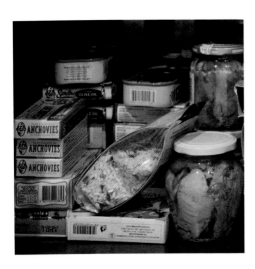

You may notice that I include anchovies quite a bit in my recipes, particularly as an added flavoring. A lot of people are averse to the strong taste of anchovies, but when you sauté them in hot oil, they dissolve, and you get a wonderful, light flavor of the sea. You don't even know anchovies are there. Many chefs use this same method of melting them down so that you are unaware you're eating them. I urge you to give them a try for the tremendous flavor they add—plus, you get the benefits of healthy omega-3 fats.

Risotto with Spring Peas

 B babies **K** kids

The trick to risotto is paying attention and making sure the rice never sticks to the pot. Double, triple, quadruple this recipe to share it with the entire family. You can also make it using frozen peeled fava beans instead of peas—everything else is the same.

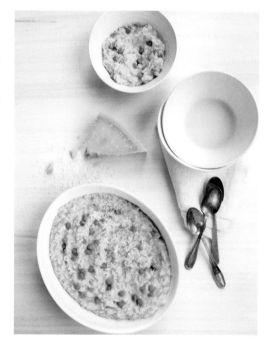

SERVES 2

4 cups chicken or vegetable stock, plus more as needed

¼ teaspoon salt, if using fresh peas

1½ cups fresh or thawed frozen spring peas

3 tablespoons extra-virgin olive oil

2 tablespoons chopped shallot or yellow onion

2 heaping handfuls dried risotto rice (see Note), such as Arborio

4 tablespoons white wine, optional (if making for adults)

1 tablespoon butter (I think this is the only tablespoon of butter in this whole book!)

4 tablespoons grated Parmigiano cheese

1. Warm the stock in a medium pot over low heat.

2. If using fresh peas, bring a small pot of water to a boil with the salt and blanch the peas for 5 to 7 minutes. Drain.

3. Puree half of the peas in a blender (you can add a little stock to adjust the consistency)—this will turn the risotto green—and leave half of them whole. Set both aside.

4. Put the olive oil in a medium pan over medium heat, add the shallot, and sauté for 2 to 3 minutes.

5. Add the risotto rice, stirring it to coat with the oil.

6. Add the wine now, if you're using it. As soon as the alcohol disappears, ladle in just enough of the stock to keep the rice moist.

7. Cook the rice over medium heat until it is tender, constantly stirring and constantly adding a little more of the stock, approximately 20 minutes. You don't want it to stick to the pot.

8. About 15 minutes into the cooking time, add the whole and the pureed peas and stir.

9. At 20 minutes, shut off the heat and stir in the butter and cheese. You'll get a beautiful green creamy mixture. Depending on the consistency you want, you can add stock until it suits you.

NOTE: Dried rice expands to three times its size after it absorbs the cooking liquid.

Fish and Other Seafood

Ⓑ babies

Ⓚ kids

Ⓢ seniors

Flounder with Potatoes and Zucchini

Ⓚ kids

SERVES 4

2 teaspoons salt

10 fingerling potatoes, skin on

2 tablespoons Dijon mustard

3 tablespoons red wine vinegar

5 to 6 cornichons, finely
  chopped

2 tablespoons capers, drained

10 tablespoons extra-virgin olive
  oil

2 teaspoons black pepper

2 pounds skinless flounder fillets

3 tablespoons canola oil

3 tablespoons finely chopped
  shallots

2 medium zucchini, cut into
  strips 2 inches long and
  ¼ inch square (about 2 cups)

1. Preheat the oven to 200°F.

2. To a pot of cold water, add 1 teaspoon of the salt and the potatoes and cook over high heat for 12 to 15 minutes, until the potatoes are fork-tender but still firm.

3. Meanwhile, in a small bowl, combine the mustard, vinegar, cornichons, and capers with 4 tablespoons of the olive oil, ½ teaspoon of the salt, and 1 teaspoon of the pepper. Mix well and set this sauce aside.

4. Season the flounder with the remaining ½ teaspoon of salt and 1 teaspoon of pepper.

5. In a large pan, heat the canola oil and 3 tablespoons of olive oil over high heat until it just begins to smoke.

6. Add the fish fillets and sauté them on medium to high heat for 3 minutes; gently flip and sauté them for another 2 to 3 minutes. Remove the fish and keep them warm in the oven.

7. Slice the potatoes ¼ inch thick and add them to the hot pan along with the remaining 3 tablespoons of olive oil, the shallots, and the zucchini. Sauté for 3 to 4 minutes.

8. Place the fillets on a large serving platter along with the vegetables and top the fish with the sauce.

Broiled Mackerel Fillets with Salt

If you're not familiar with mackerel, this recipe is a great place to start, as this is a really tasty, simple dish. Plan ahead, as you'll need to put the fillets in the refrigerator for 1 to 2 hours before cooking them. It's even better if you allow them to chill overnight. The yield for this recipe is actually double the amount I need for a meal. That's because I make extra and put what's left over in the fridge. The next day I'll make a salad out of it—see my directions below.

SERVES 8

8 mackerel fillets (4 to 6 ounces each)

1 tablespoon salt

5 tablespoons extra-virgin olive oil

1 lemon, cut into wedges

1. On the skin side, score the mackerel diagonally, 2 to 3 slices per fillet, cutting just deeply enough to reach the meat.

2. Salt the fish on both sides and refrigerate for 1 to 2 hours or overnight.

3. Prepare the oven to broil and place the rack 4 inches from the heat source. Oil a baking pan with 1 tablespoon of the oil.

4. Shake off the excess salt from the fish, drizzle both sides with 2 tablespoons of the olive oil, and place them on the prepared baking pan skin side up (or else the fish will dry out).

5. Broil the mackerel for 3 to 4 minutes, until it is dark golden, taking care not to overcook it, as mackerel cooks quickly.

6. Place the mackerel on a serving platter, skin facing up, and serve the fillets with wedges of lemon. Drizzle the fish with the remaining 2 tablespoons of oil.

> **SALAD OPTION:** Break up 4 leftover mackerel fillets into small pieces, making sure to remove the skin and bones. Place it in a bowl. Add ½ teaspoon salt, ½ teaspoon black pepper, 1 tablespoon red wine vinegar, juice of ½ lemon, ¼ cup chopped celery, ½ medium onion (chopped), 2 tablespoons capers (drained and chopped), 3 tablespoons extra-virgin olive oil, and 1 heaping tablespoon mayonnaise.

Red Snapper alla Palermitana

This is the way they prepare red snapper in the capital city of Sicily.

SERVES 4

8 tablespoons extra-virgin olive
   oil

1 medium onion, thinly sliced

2 medium Yukon Gold potatoes,
   peeled and thinly sliced

1 tablespoon fresh rosemary,
   chopped

1 teaspoon ground red pepper
   flakes (see Note)

1½ teaspoons salt

½ cup flour

2 (1½- to 2-pound) red
   snappers, scaled and cleaned

1 cup marsala wine

Juice of 1 lemon

1. Preheat the oven to 375°F.

2. Put 4 tablespoons of the oil in a large pan over low heat, and add the onion. Sauté for 2 minutes (do not let the onion turn color).

3. Add the potatoes, rosemary, red pepper, and ½ teaspoon of the salt. Sauté for 3 to 5 minutes and set aside.

4. In a shallow bowl, stir together the flour and the remaining 1 teaspoon of salt. Dredge the fish in the mixture.

5. Put 3 tablespoons of the oil in a large oven-safe pan over medium-high heat. Sauté the floured fish for 1 minute on each side.

6. Add the marsala and lemon juice to the pan and allow it to reduce by half.

7. Add the potatoes and onion to the fish and transfer the pan to the oven. After 10 minutes, turn the fish once and stir the potatoes and onion two or three times. Continue baking for 5 minutes longer.

8. Serve the fish with the potatoes and onion, with the pan juices poured over the top.

NOTE: I use a spice grinder to grind red pepper flakes into a fine powder. In a pinch, you can use them whole.

Calamari e Piselli
(Sautéed Calamari and Peas)

Squid requires additional prep work, but it's worth it! See my tips on buying, storing, and cooking squid starting on page 92.

SERVES 4

¼ cup extra-virgin olive oil

¼ cup finely chopped onion

½ teaspoon red pepper flakes

1 tablespoon chopped garlic

2 tablespoons chopped fresh
   parsley

1 cup crushed plum tomatoes
   (I do this by hand), juice
   reserved

2 pounds medium-size squid,
   cut into rings and tentacles,
   thoroughly cleaned

1 cup frozen peas, thawed

1 teaspoon salt

1 teaspoon black pepper

1. Put the oil in a large pan over medium heat. Add the onion and red pepper flakes, and cook until the onion becomes soft. Add the garlic and sauté for 1 minute.

2. Stir in the parsley and tomatoes with their juice; cover and simmer for 8 to 10 minutes.

3. Add the squid, cover the pan, and simmer on low heat (see Note) for 15 minutes, stirring occasionally.

4. Add the peas, salt, and pepper, and cook for 5 minutes more. Serve hot.

> NOTE: When cooking squid or mussels, always cook over low heat.

Broiled Halibut Salad

This recipe features a fillet of halibut topped with a fresh mixed salad. Dryer fish like halibut is often well accompanied by a succulent topping.

SERVES 4

4 cloves garlic, finely minced
1½ teaspoons salt
3 tablespoons extra-virgin olive oil

Two 1-pound halibut fillets, 1-inch thick

SALAD

¾ cup grape tomatoes, halved
½ red onion, thinly sliced
3 tablespoons extra-virgin olive oil
½ teaspoon salt
½ teaspoon black pepper
¼ cup Kalamata olives, pitted and sliced

1 teaspoon roughly chopped cilantro
¼ cup chopped seeded cucumber
½ tablespoon red wine vinegar

1. Prepare the oven to broil. Combine the minced garlic, salt, and oil in a medium bowl.

2. Coat each side of the fish fillets with the seasoned oil and place them on an oiled baking pan.

3. Broil the fish for 3 to 4 minutes on each side. Be careful not to overcook it; halibut should be moist when served.

4. To make the salad accompaniment, combine all the salad ingredients in a bowl, and spoon the mixture on top of the halibut steaks before serving.

Baked Orata

Orata (also known as bream and dorado) is found in the Mediterranean Sea and the eastern coastal regions of the North Atlantic Ocean. It's a flaky white fish with a slightly sweet flavor, and the tender flesh is often used in stews like bouillabaisse because it doesn't fall apart when cooked. Orata also provides healthy omega-3 fats, is low in environmental mercury, and is budget-friendly. When shopping for it, look for firmness, clear eyes, and a sea smell.

SERVES 2

3 tablespoons extra-virgin olive oil

1 large Yukon Gold or russet potato, cut into ¼-inch-thick slices

¾ teaspoon salt

¼ cup white wine

20 Kalamata olives, pitted and halved

2 tablespoons capers

1 tablespoon fresh rosemary, chopped

2 (1½- to 2-pound) orata, scaled and cleaned

½ teaspoon black pepper

1. Preheat the oven to 400°F. Oil a rimmed baking pan.

2. Put 2 tablespoons of the oil in a large pan over medium heat. Add the potatoes and ¼ teaspoon of the salt, and sauté for 3 to 4 minutes.

3. Add the wine, olives, capers, and rosemary, partially cover the pan, and cook for another 2 to 3 minutes.

4. Arrange the orata in the prepared baking pan. Drizzle them with the remaining 1 tablespoon of oil and sprinkle on both sides with ½ teaspoon each of salt and pepper. Bake the fish for 7 minutes.

5. Turn the fish over and add the potato-olive-caper mixture; bake for another 5 minutes.

6. Plate the fish and spoon the juice and potato-olive-caper mixture over the fish.

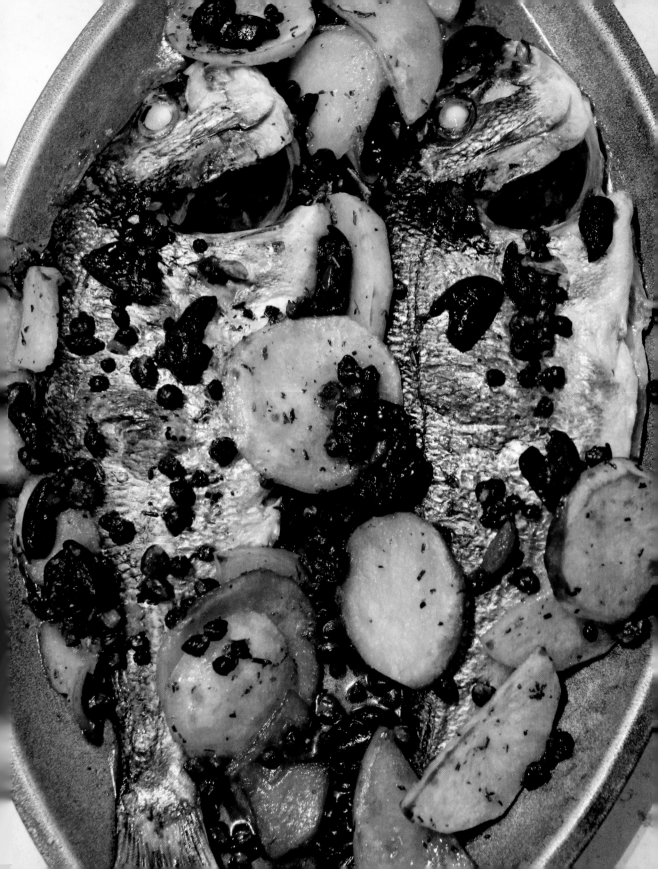

Baked Swordfish Milanese

SERVES 4

8 tablespoons extra-virgin olive oil

1½ cups panko bread crumbs

1½ pounds swordfish, cut into
    ¼-inch-thick cutlet slices

1 teaspoon salt

1 teaspoon black pepper

About ¾ cup Simple Bruschetta
    topping (see page 188)

1. Preheat the oven to 425°F.

2. Pour 6 tablespoons of the olive oil into a shallow dish. Place the bread crumbs into a resealable plastic bag and lightly crush them into a slightly finer consistency, which will help them to better stick to the swordfish. Place the bread crumbs in a separate shallow dish.

3. Sprinkle the fish with the salt and pepper. Dredge the fish on both sides, first in oil, then in the bread crumbs.

4. Coat the bottom of a nonstick baking pan with the remaining 2 tablespoons of oil and place the fish slices in the pan in a single layer. Bake them for 4 minutes, turn them over, then increase the oven temperature to broil them for 30 seconds.

5. Top each serving with about 2 tablespoons of the bruschetta topping before serving.

Fish Substitutions

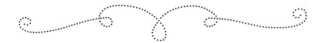

When you can't find a certain fish called for in my recipes, or it's not looking very fresh, try one of these substitutions (cooking times may differ):

Flounder = Sole

Tilefish = Cod, halibut

Red snapper = Striped bass, black bass,
    tilapia, porgy

Halibut = Cod, tilefish

Orata = Branzino, red snapper, black sea
    bass, striped bass

Langoustine = Lobster

Mussels = Clams (sometimes)

Lemon sole = Regular sole, flounder

Chilean sea bass = Cod

Branzino = Striped bass, black bass,
    red snapper, orata

Swordfish = Tuna

Mussels with Tomatoes

What I remember most about growing up in Sicily is that almost all of the dishes contained garlic and tomatoes. This recipe is a variation on steamed mussels that I like because you can dunk bread into the broth, which turns it into an entire meal. See my tips on buying, storing, and cooking mussels beginning on page 92.

SERVES 4

3 tablespoons extra-virgin olive oil

1 large onion, chopped

4 cloves garlic, crushed

1 teaspoon salt

1 teaspoon red pepper flakes

8 fresh or canned plum tomatoes, roughly chopped

6 pounds mussels, washed and scrubbed

10 leaves fresh basil, roughly chopped

⅔ cup white wine

Loaf of Italian baguette

1. Put the oil in a large, wide pot over medium heat. Add the onion, garlic, salt, and red pepper flakes. Sauté until the onion is soft.

2. Add the tomatoes, cover, and cook for 20 minutes.

3. Puree the tomato mixture in batches, using a blender.

4. Transfer the puree back to the pot, add the mussels, basil, and wine, and cook over low to medium heat, covered, for 3 to 6 minutes, stirring occasionally. Discard any mussels that haven't opened after 6 minutes.

5. Serve with plenty of sliced bread on the table.

Tuna alla Siciliana

SERVES 6

½ cup extra-virgin olive oil

3 cloves garlic, sliced

8 to 10 fresh mint leaves

2 pounds tuna steaks, 1-inch
    thick

1½ teaspoons salt

1 teaspoon black pepper

½ cup white wine

1 medium onion, chopped

1 pound tomatoes, peeled,
    seeded, and chopped

1. In a large pan, heat ¼ cup of the oil over medium heat. Add the garlic and mint, and sauté for 30 seconds. Season the tuna with ½ teaspoon of the salt, add the steaks to the pan, and sauté for 1 minute on each side. Remove the tuna steaks and set them aside so that they don't continue to cook.

2. Add ½ teaspoon each of the salt and pepper to the pan, as well as the wine, and cook for another 2 to 3 minutes, until the wine is reduced by half. Remove the pan from the heat and set it aside.

3. In another pan over medium heat, put the remaining ¼ cup oil; add the onion and sauté until it softens.

4. Add the chopped tomatoes and the remaining ½ teaspoon each of salt and pepper to the onion. Cook for 5 to 7 minutes more.

5. Return the tuna to the pan with the wine reduction. Add the tomato and onion mixture to the tuna, then stir in ½ cup of very hot water. Cover the pan and cook over medium heat for 3 minutes more.

6. Remove the pan from the heat, and slice the tuna. Pour the sauce from the pan over the top and serve.

Spaghetti with Fresh Tuna and Thyme

S seniors

This recipe features a quick sauce that can be made while the pasta is cooking.

SERVES 6

1 tablespoon plus 1 teaspoon
  salt
1 pound spaghetti
½ cup extra-virgin olive oil
1 medium onion, finely chopped
4 anchovies in oil, chopped
1 teaspoon red pepper flakes

1 pound fresh tuna, cut into
  ½-inch cubes
¼ cup white wine
2 plum tomatoes, peeled,
  seeded, and chopped
1 tablespoon fresh thyme,
  chopped

1. Bring a large pot of water to boil over high heat. Add 1 tablespoon of the salt and the pasta, and cook according to the package instructions until al dente.

2. Meanwhile, put ¼ cup of the oil in a large pan over low to medium heat. Add the onion, anchovies, and red pepper flakes and cook for 4 to 5 minutes. Add 1 to 2 tablespoons of water, a tablespoon at a time, if needed to prevent the onion from burning.

3. When the onion softens up, raise the heat to medium-high, add the tuna and the remaining 1 teaspoon of salt and cook for 30 seconds, stirring. You want to just sear the tuna, not cook it all the way through.

4. Add the wine and tomatoes, stir, and cook for another minute, then stir in the thyme.

5. Drain the pasta, then immediately add it to the pan and cook the mixture for another half minute.

6. Stir in the remaining ¼ cup of oil and serve.

Sicilian Seafood Paella

This decorative and delicious dish sounds complicated, but it takes only one to two pans, cooks fast, makes for an easy cleanup, and is a crowd-pleaser. Note that cooking the mussels and clams separately as I suggest in my recipe is a good way to control the optimal preparation, as mussels and clams cook at different rates.

SERVES 8

¼ cup extra-virgin olive oil
1 large onion, chopped
3 cloves garlic, finely chopped
1 red bell pepper, seeded and sliced
1 green bell pepper, seeded and sliced
2 cups long-grain rice
1 teaspoon salt
1½ teaspoons saffron threads
½ cup white wine
1 quart fresh clam juice (or canned or bottled clam juice or fish stock)

1 pound cleaned squid, cut into ½-inch rings
2 dozen littleneck clams, scrubbed with a small brush to get the sand off
1 pound mussels, cleaned by rubbing them together in your hands under cold running water
½ pound medium shrimp, peeled and deveined
½ pound dry scallops
1 cup frozen peas, thawed

1. Put the oil in a large paella pan (or a very large sauté pan) over low to medium heat. Add the onion, garlic, and 1 to 2 tablespoons water (to keep the onion from burning) and sauté until the onion is soft.

2. Add the peppers to the pan and sauté for another 3 minutes while stirring.

3. Stir in the rice, coating it with the olive oil, and add the salt and saffron.

4. Add the wine and cook for 2 to 3 minutes more.

5. Add the clam juice. Turn the heat to high, and when the mixture starts to boil, reduce the heat to maintain a simmer.

6. Stir in the squid. Stir occasionally to prevent sticking (some say not to stir, but usually paella pans are not good enough and everything sticks) and cook for 15 to 20 minutes.

7. In a large pot, combine the clams and 2 tablespoons of water over medium

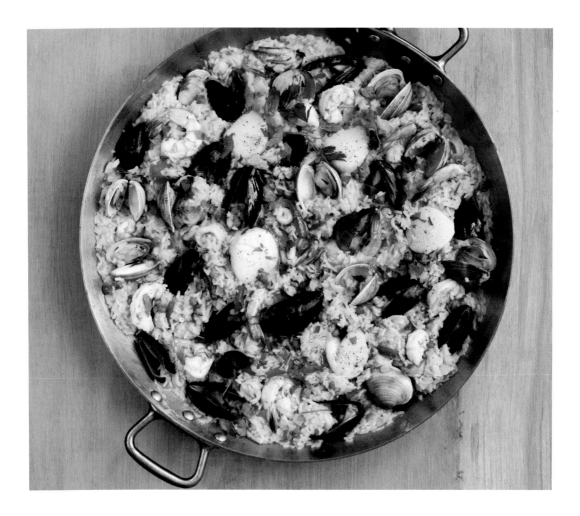

heat, put the cover on, and cook until they just open, about 3 to 5 minutes—don't overcook or they'll get tough and rubbery. Transfer the clams and their juice to a large bowl.

8. Add the mussels and 2 tablespoons of water to the same pot, and cook them over medium heat as you cooked the clams—the mussels will take only 2 to 3 minutes to open. Add the mussels and their cooking liquid to the bowl with the clams.

9. Strain the juice from the clams and mussels and add it to the paella pan.

10. After the rice has been cooking for 15 minutes, add the shrimp, scallops, and peas to the paella pan, stir, and allow the paella to cook for 4 to 5 minutes. The shrimp and scallops are fully cooked when they become opaque white.

11. Place the clams and mussels on top of the mixture in the paella pan and serve.

Lemon Sole

Ⓚ kids

Lemon sole is a more delicate (and more expensive) kind of sole. You can use regular sole in this recipe, but I like lemon sole for introducing kids to fish because it's not very "fishy"—it doesn't have a strong smell or taste of fish. For adults, I love topping each slice of sole fillet with 2 tablespoons of my tomato bruschetta mixture (see page 188).

SERVES 4

4 slices of lemon sole (or sole)
1 teaspoon salt
8 tablespoons extra-virgin olive
    oil

About ¾ cup all-purpose flour,
    for dredging

1. Sprinkle the fish with the salt.

2. Put 6 tablespoons of the olive oil in a skillet over medium to high heat.

3. Dredge the slices of sole in the flour and gently sauté them for 2 minutes on each side.

4. Remove the fish from the pan.

5. For children's servings, using a fork, mash each fillet with some of the remaining 1 tablespoon of olive oil. For adults, drizzle the remaining olive oil over the intact fillets.

Chilean Sea Bass with Tomatoes, Capers, and Olives

You can also use another firm white fish in this recipe, such as striped sea bass or grouper.

SERVES 4 TO 6

6 plum tomatoes
9 tablespoons extra-virgin olive
   oil
4 cloves garlic, crushed
Salt
¼ cup white wine
3 tablespoons capers, drained
20 Sicilian green olives, pitted
   and quartered

Black pepper
1½ pounds Chilean sea bass, cut
   into 4 to 6 serving portions
¼ cup flour (Wondra quick-
   mixing flour preferred)
¼ cup coarsely chopped fresh
   basil

1. Preheat the oven to 400°F.

2. Bring a large pot of water to a boil over high heat. Cut an X in the bottom of each plum tomato, blanch the tomatoes for 1 minute in the boiling water, then remove them. Peel and seed the tomatoes and cut them into quarters.

3. Put 4 tablespoons of the olive oil in a large pan over medium heat; add the garlic and cook until it turns golden. Add the tomatoes, ½ teaspoon of salt, and the white wine. Simmer for 1 minute—you don't want to cook this for too long. Add the capers and olives and cook for 2 more minutes. Remove the pan from the heat and set it aside.

4. Put 3 tablespoons of the olive oil in an oven-safe pan over medium heat. Salt and pepper the fish and dredge it in the flour.

5. Once the oil is hot, add the fish pieces and sauté on each side for 30 seconds, then place the pan in the oven for 6 to 7 minutes, uncovered.

6. Carefully remove the pan from the oven. Pour the tomato mixture on top (it will sizzle) and spread it evenly. Sprinkle with the basil and drizzle the remaining 2 tablespoons of olive oil over the dish just before serving.

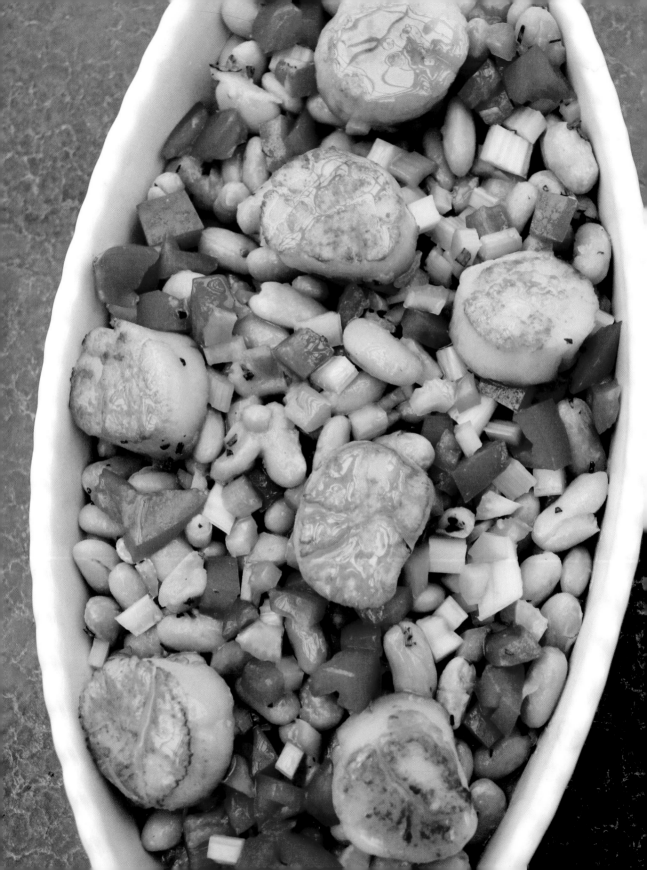

Scallops with Cannellini Beans

This recipe is versatile, as you can make a variety of substitutions: try swapping shrimp for the scallops and chickpeas for the cannellini beans. You can also use thyme for the herb instead of rosemary.

For convenience, you can do much in advance, preparing the whole dish except for the celery and tomatoes, then warming everything up and adding the celery and tomatoes just before serving. Note that if you use dried cannellini beans, they'll need to soak overnight beforehand.

SERVES 4 TO 6 AS AN APPETIZER, OR 2 TO 3 AS A MAIN COURSE

1¼ cups dried cannellini beans, soaked overnight and drained, or 2½ (14- to 16-ounce) cans cannellini beans, drained

Salt

8 to 12 large dry scallops, muscle/tendon removed (see page 94)

Black pepper

8 tablespoons extra-virgin olive oil

3 cloves garlic, crushed

¼ cup dry white wine

1 teaspoon chopped fresh rosemary

1 teaspoon red pepper flakes

¼ cup chopped celery, optional

2 tomatoes, seeded and chopped into ¼-inch cubes, optional

1. If you're using dried cannellini beans, after soaking and draining them, cook them in a pot of boiling water over medium-high heat for approximately 1 hour until tender. After they have cooked, stir 1 tablespoon of salt into the pot, then drain the beans and set them aside. (You add the salt at this point because they are hard and impenetrable until they're cooked to tenderness.)

2. If you are using canned beans, drain them from their juice; some, especially those who are watching their sodium intake, should also rinse, but I don't, because I like the thickness the unrinsed beans add to the sauce. Make sure the scallops are nice and dry and salt and pepper them to taste. Place a nonstick frying pan over medium heat, coat the bottom with 3 tablespoons of the oil, and

continued >

when the oil is hot, add the garlic and cook until it turns golden. Remove the garlic from the oil.

3. Turn up the heat, and just before the oil starts to smoke (it has to be very hot), add the scallops, taking care not to crowd the pan. Cook each scallop for 2 minutes, 1 minute for each side. When you turn the scallops over after the first minute of sautéing, add the wine, then, when the scallops are done, remove them from the frying pan and set them aside.

4. In the same pan, add 3 tablespoons of the olive oil, and after the oil is heated, add the cannellini beans (if you're using canned beans, add ½ teaspoon of salt here), rosemary, and red pepper flakes. Sauté for about 2 minutes. Then return the scallops, along with their juices, to the pan and let them cook for another 1 to 2 minutes together.

5. Take the pan off the heat, and for a crunchy touch, if desired, stir in the celery and tomatoes.

6. Spoon cannellini beans onto each plate and place 2 scallops on top for an appetizer portion and 4 scallops for a main course. Drizzle with the remaining 2 tablespoons of olive oil and serve immediately so the celery and tomato don't cook and lose their crunch.

Tuna Tartare

Since this dish involves raw tuna, you must get fresh, high-quality, sushi-grade tuna ("sushi-grade" is not officially regulated, but it should mean that the fish is free of parasites that can make you sick and is safe to eat raw). Go to a fishmonger you trust, one with a clean environment and healthful food practices. Tuna may be treated with carbon monoxide gas to brighten and redden its color, so it's important to have a trustworthy fish source. (The treatment is generally regarded as safe, but could mask the age and quality of the tuna.) The tuna should be bright red. If it's very red or brown, it may be past its prime and no good.

You also don't want to use tuna that has a lot of white fiber in it. When you get a chunk, look at the core, and if you see white fibrous material toward the outside of the fish, cut it off.

SERVES 6

1 pound sushi-grade tuna, cut into ¼-inch cubes
1 teaspoon Dijon mustard
1 teaspoon salt
1 teaspoon black pepper
2 tablespoons sesame oil (not toasted)

2 tablespoons capers, drained and chopped
2 tablespoons chopped shallots
3 tablespoons peeled, seeded, and chopped cucumber
1 tablespoon finely chopped fresh ginger

1. In a large bowl, gently mix all of the ingredients with your hands.

2. Place a round metal cookie cutter on a plate, put 3 to 4 tablespoons of the mixture in it, and gently press with the bottom of a spoon to mold the portion.

3. Remove the metal circle and serve cold.

Branzini all' Acqua Pazza with Clams and Mussels

Branzino, a sea bass native to the East Atlantic and Mediterranean Sea, ranges in size from 1½ to 3 pounds and has firm, white, delicate-flavored meat with few small bones. It's rich in omega-3 fats, protein, and the antioxidant selenium. Farm-raised branzino is low in environmental mercury.

SERVES 4

2 branzini (1½ to 2 pounds each), filleted (4 fillets)
½ teaspoon salt
1 teaspoon black pepper
6 tablespoons extra-virgin olive oil
6 cloves garlic, crushed
1 tablespoon tomato paste

⅓ cup white wine
1 dozen littleneck clams, washed and scrubbed
2 pounds mussels, washed and scrubbed
1 to 2 tablespoons chopped fresh parsley, for garnish

1. Sprinkle the fillets on the flesh side with the salt and pepper.

2. Heat a sauté pan over medium-high heat. Add 4 tablespoons of the olive oil, the garlic cloves, and tomato paste and sauté until the garlic is golden. Add the wine and layer the fish fillets on top of the garlic.

3. Stand the clams on the sides of the pan, with the muscle end (where they connect) against the edges of the pan. Cover the pan and cook on medium heat for about 4 minutes.

4. Uncover, add the mussels, cover again, and cook for another 3 minutes, until the mussels open.

5. Remove the pan from the heat. Discard any mussels and clams that haven't opened and drizzle the remaining 2 tablespoons of olive oil over the fish. Garnish with the parsley and spoon the pan juices over the fish as you're serving.

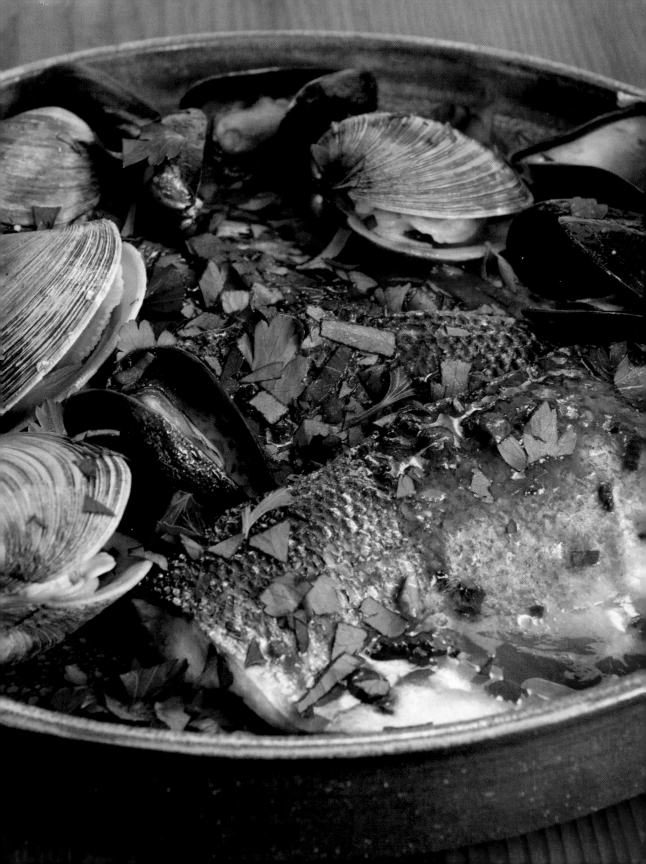

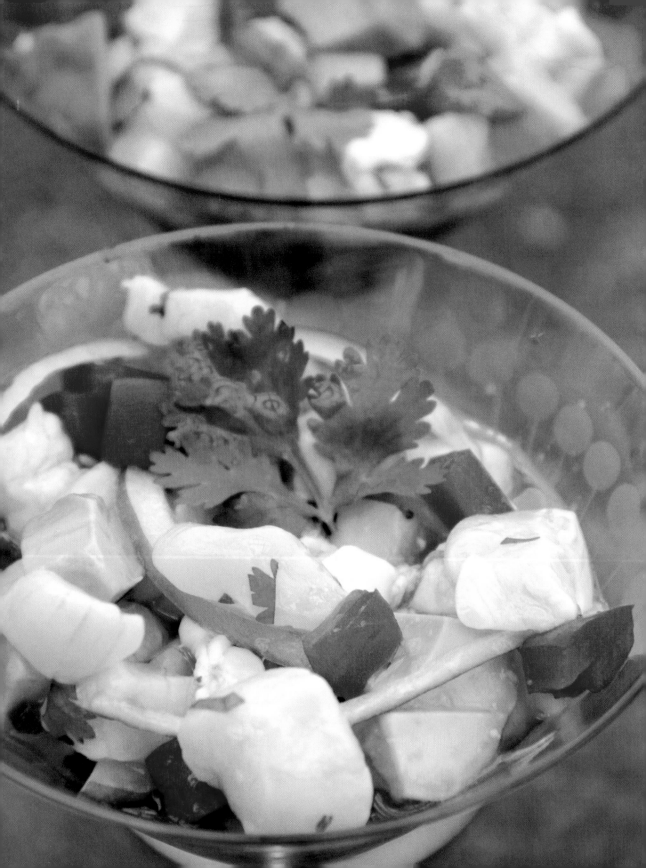

Halibut and Scallop Ceviche

This chilled seafood dish is especially terrific on a warm summer night. Not only is it delicious, but it packs in a variety of Mediterranean superstars—omega-3 fat from the avocado and two varieties of seafood; citrus, tomatoes, and onions bursting with antioxidants and polyphenols; as well as fresh, uncooked olive oil.

SERVES 4

½ pound halibut, cut into ⅓-inch cubes

½ pound bay scallops

½ red onion, thinly sliced

½ teaspoon salt

1 jalapeño pepper, seeded and finely chopped

Juice of 1 lemon

Juice of 1 orange

Juice of 2 limes

1 tablespoon chopped fresh cilantro leaves

Flesh of 1 avocado, cut into ⅓-inch cubes

2 plum tomatoes, seeded and cut into ⅓-inch cubes

2 tablespoons extra-virgin olive oil (see Note)

1. In a bowl, combine the halibut, scallops, onion, salt, jalapeño, and citrus juices. Marinate the mixture in the refrigerator for 30 minutes.
2. Mix in the cilantro, avocado, and tomatoes.
3. Serve in a martini glass, drizzled with the olive oil (see Note).

NOTE: You may have noticed that even though I cook with olive oil as I'm preparing a dish, I often drizzle fresh olive oil over it just before I serve it. That's because uncooked oil has a different flavor than cooked oil, and I like the savory essence the fresh oil brings. The olive oil I add in the end is also the healthiest, as oxidational power can be lost during the cooking process.

Salmon with Orange and Lemon

This variation of the salmon recipe in my book *The Mediterranean Prescription* was suggested by my wife, Svetlana. Many children find this recipe tasty; however, it does contain honey, which should be left out for those under a year old, even when cooked.

This dish is best if the salmon is left to marinate for an hour and a half before cooking.

SERVES 4 TO 6

Juice of 2 oranges
Juice of 1½ lemons
2 tablespoons soy sauce
2 tablespoons honey, optional
3 tablespoons extra-virgin olive
   oil, plus extra if desired

2 pounds skin-on salmon fillet
½ teaspoon salt
½ teaspoon black pepper,
   optional

1. In a large baking dish, combine the orange and lemon juices, soy sauce, honey (if using), and olive oil. Stir the mixture to dissolve the honey.

2. Season the salmon on both sides with the salt (and pepper if for adults only).

3. Add the salmon to the juice mixture and marinate it in the refrigerator for 45 minutes per side.

4. Prepare the oven to broil.

5. Place the salmon under the broiler, skin side down, and cook it for 10 to 12 minutes, depending on the thickness.

6. For young children, mash the fish with a fork and add extra olive oil to make it creamy. Serve the soft inner meat to those who like a smoother texture (don't forgo broiling or the flavor suffers). Spoon the cooked juice from the baking dish over the salmon and serve immediately.

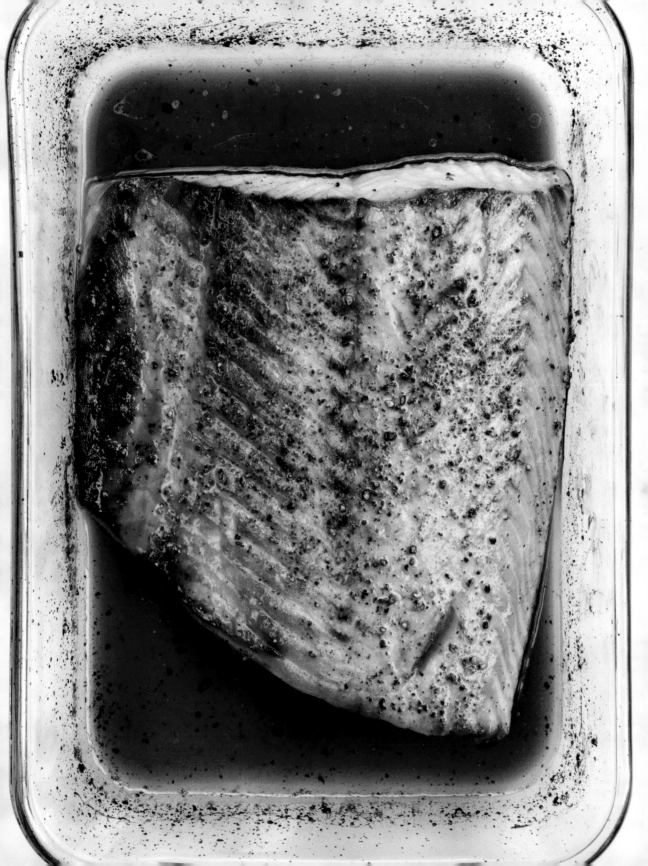

Poultry and Meat

Ⓑ babies

Ⓚ kids

Ⓢ seniors

Chicken with Capers

SERVES 4

4 tablespoons extra-virgin olive oil

4 anchovy fillets, chopped

3 tablespoons capers

1½ pounds chicken cutlets, pounded (see Note)

½ teaspoon salt

1 teaspoon black pepper

2 cloves garlic, finely chopped

Juice of 3 lemons

3 tablespoons chopped fresh parsley

1. Put 2 tablespoons of the olive oil in a large pan over medium heat. Add the anchovies and the capers and, with a wooden spoon, mash the anchovies into the oil until they dissolve, about 2 minutes.

2. Sprinkle the chicken cutlets with the salt and pepper, push aside the capers, and place the cutlets in the pan.

3. Sauté the chicken cutlets on each side for about 2 minutes, until cooked through.

4. Remove the cutlets, add the garlic, and cook it for 20 to 30 seconds. Deglaze the pan with two-thirds of the lemon juice.

5. Return the cutlets to the pan for another 30 seconds, mixing them with the cooking juices.

6. Remove the cutlets from the pan and spoon capers and juice on top. Drizzle them with the remaining 2 tablespoons of oil and the remaining lemon juice, and sprinkle with parsley.

NOTE: A problem with chicken breasts and cutlets is that their thickness is often uneven, so the meat cooks unevenly. To rectify this, pound breasts or cutlets between two sheets of plastic wrap or in a plastic zip-top bag using a meat mallet or heavy pan until the whole piece is an even ½-inch thickness.

Yogurt-Marinated Chicken

The reason many Middle Eastern countries and southern Italian cultur͏ nate their chicken in yogurt is that it moistens and tenderizes the chicken. If you set some of the yogurt mixture aside before you marinate it, it will make a delicious accompaniment after the chicken is prepared.

SERVES 4

3 limes

3 tablespoons extra-virgin olive oil, plus more for drizzling

2 cloves garlic, finely chopped

20 leaves fresh basil, chopped

3 tablespoons chopped chives

1 tablespoon black pepper

1½ cups yogurt

1 teaspoon salt

2 tablespoons chopped scallions

1 chicken, cut into 8 pieces

Sliced scallions, for garnish

1. Set one of the limes aside to use for garnish. From the remaining limes, grate 1 tablespoon of zest; squeeze the juice from 2 of the limes.

2. Put the lime zest and juice in a blender, along with the oil, garlic, basil, chives, pepper, yogurt, salt, and chopped scallions. Puree to a smooth marinade. Reserve and refrigerate ⅓ cup of the marinade.

3. Pour the remaining marinade into a large bowl and add the chicken quarters, tossing them to coat. Cover and refrigerate the bowl, and let the meat marinate for approximately 8 hours.

4. Preheat the oven to 475°F. Cut the reserved lime into wedges. Allow the reserved marinade to come to room temperature.

5. Remove the chicken from the marinade, shake it off, pat it dry, and drizzle it with oil.

6. Place the chicken on a baking sheet and bake it for approximately 40 minutes.

7. Serve the chicken with the reserved marinade and wedges of lime alongside, and garnished with sliced scallions.

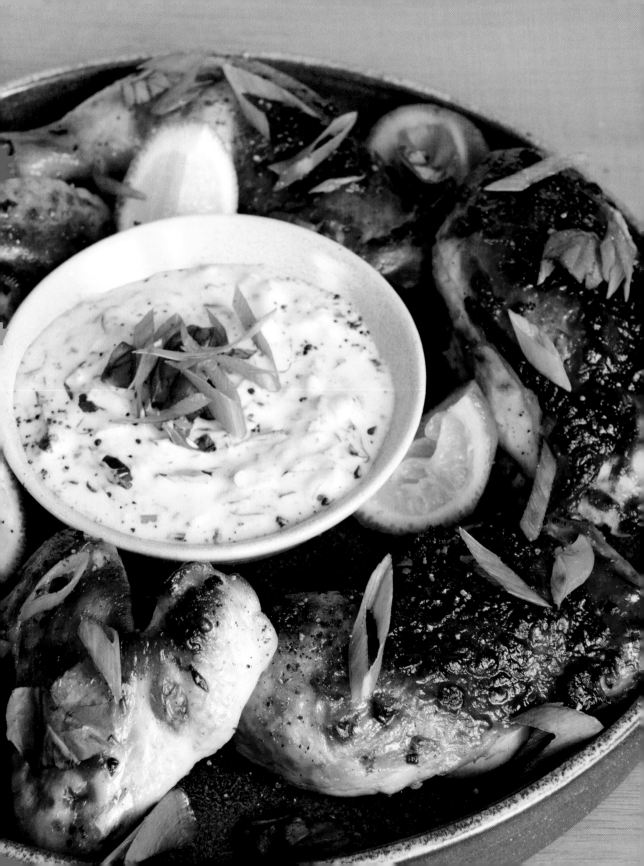

Lime-Marinated Chicken Thighs

K kids

This recipe was given to me by my business partner, Dr. Diego Diaz. It has become one of my children's favorites. Whenever we go to the country we barbecue this. The meat is moist and has a wonderful, balanced flavor.

SERVES 4

2 pounds chicken thighs
1 teaspoon salt
1 teaspoon black pepper
7 limes, 6 juiced and 1 cut into
  wedges for serving

3 tablespoons canola oil
1 tablespoon extra-virgin olive oil

1. Combine the chicken, salt, pepper, lime juice, and canola oil in a resealable plastic bag. Refrigerate and let the meat marinate for 4 hours.

2. Prepare the oven to broil.

3. Remove the thighs from the marinade, shake off the excess liquid, and place them on a baking pan. Broil them for 4 to 5 minutes on each side.

4. Serve with the lime wedges alongside the chicken thighs. Squeeze fresh lime onto the chicken, drizzle with the olive oil, and enjoy.

Baked Chicken Tenders

....

These taste even better than the fried version! I give my kids different jobs to do after the chicken is cured, such as sprinkling salt, dredging the tenders, or drizzling them with olive oil.

SERVES 2

½ pound presliced chicken tenders or chicken cutlets cut into long strips

2 tablespoons salt, plus more as needed

3 tablespoons extra-virgin olive oil

2 cloves garlic, finely chopped

½ cup seasoned bread crumbs

2 tablespoons grated Parmigiano cheese

1. Cure the chicken by soaking it in cold water to cover with the salt for 10 to 15 minutes. Rinse the cutlets off and pat them dry.

2. In a sealed plastic bag, combine the chicken tenders with 2 tablespoons of the olive oil and the garlic. Allow them to marinate for 1 hour in the refrigerator.

3. Preheat the oven to 400°F. Coat a baking pan with olive oil.

4. Remove the chicken from the bag and shake off any excess garlic. Sprinkle it with a pinch of salt, if desired.

5. In a separate dish, mix the bread crumbs and Parmigiano cheese, and roll your chicken in it so each piece is coated.

6. Place the chicken tenders on the prepared baking pan and drizzle a little of the remaining 1 tablespoon of olive oil over each one.

7. Bake the tenders for 10 minutes, turn them over, then cook them for another 3 minutes.

Easy Baked Chicken Cutlets

K kids

These are terrific served with bruschetta toppings (see pages 188–189), about two tablespoons per cutlet. I like to pair this dish with a side of broccoli rabe or escarole salad with olive oil and white balsamic vinaigrette.

SERVES 4

1½ pounds chicken cutlets,
    evenly pounded to ½ inch
    thick
Salt
1 cup seasoned bread crumbs

¼ cup grated Parmigiano cheese
2 cloves garlic, finely chopped
1 teaspoon black pepper
¼ cup extra-virgin olive oil, plus
    more as needed

1. Cure the chicken by soaking it in enough cold water to cover, mixed with 2 tablespoons of salt, for 10 to 15 minutes. Rinse the cutlets off and pat them dry.

2. Preheat the oven to 400°F. Grease a sheet pan with olive oil.

3. Mix the bread crumbs, grated cheese, and garlic.

4. Sprinkle both sides of the chicken using 1 teaspoon each salt and pepper, then dredge both sides of the cutlets in the olive oil.

5. Coat the cutlets in the bread crumb mixture and place them on the prepared pan.

6. Drizzle the tops with ½ teaspoon olive oil and bake them for 10 to 12 minutes. Turn them over, drizzle them with olive oil, and bake for another 3 minutes.

7. Increase the oven temperature to broil, and broil the cutlets for 3 minutes to give them a nice toasty color and a little bit of crunchiness, taking care not to burn the bread crumbs (or they will turn very bitter).

Veal Cutlets Sicilian-Style

Serve this dish hot with a leafy cold salad tossed with oil and vinegar dressing.

SERVES 4

3 tablespoons white wine vinegar

1 pound veal cutlets, thinly sliced and beaten

¼ cup chopped fresh parsley

1 clove garlic, finely chopped

¼ cup grated pecorino cheese

2 eggs, beaten

½ cup plain bread crumbs

½ tablespoon salt

½ tablespoon black pepper

¼ cup extra-virgin olive oil

1. Put the vinegar and the veal cutlets in a resealable plastic bag and allow the meat to marinate for 20 minutes.

2. Prepare three bowls: in one, combine the parsley, garlic, and cheese; in the second, the beaten eggs; and in the third, the bread crumbs.

3. Remove the cutlets from the bag, shake off the vinegar, and sprinkle both sides with the salt and pepper.

4. Dredge the cutlets on both sides in the cheese mixture, then wet both sides with egg, and finish by coating both sides in the bread crumbs.

5. Pour the oil into a large pot over high heat. Just before the oil begins to smoke, add the breaded veal and cook for 40 to 60 seconds per side. Drain the cutlets on a paper-towel-lined plate before serving.

Marinated Pork Tenderloin

Brussels sprouts, sautéed kale, broccoli rabe, and grilled potatoes all go very well with this dish.

SERVES 6

2 pork tenderloins, about 1 to 1½ pounds each

½ cup lemon juice

6 cloves garlic, chopped

2 tablespoons chopped fresh rosemary

2 tablespoons chopped fresh thyme

1 teaspoon salt

1 tablespoon Dijon mustard

⅓ cup extra-virgin olive oil

1 tablespoon brown sugar

1. Place the pork tenderloins in a resealable plastic bag.

2. In a bowl, mix the remaining ingredients and add the marinade to the plastic bag with the pork tenderloins. Marinate overnight.

3. Preheat the oven to 425°F.

4. Remove the tenderloins from the marinade and place them in a large oven-safe pan over medium to high heat.

5. Brown the tenderloins on all sides, 1 minute on each side.

6. Transfer the pan to the oven for 10 minutes and cook until an instant-read thermometer inserted into the thickest part of a tenderloin reads 145°F.

7. Let rest for 10 minutes, then cut the tenderloin into ½-inch slices and serve 3 to 4 slices per plate.

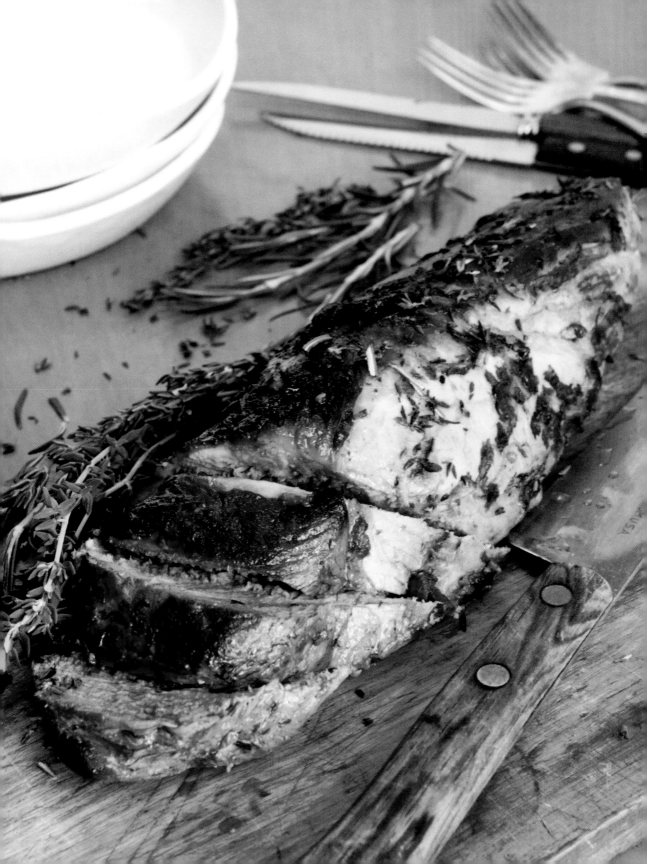

Incorporating the
Mediterranean Lifestyle at Mealtime

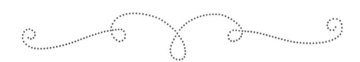

- Eat lunch outdoors at a nearby park.
- Use part of your lunch hour to take a stroll with a friend.
- Stop by the local farmers' market for groceries.
- Cook a meal with friends or the whole family helping.

- Turn off all electronics during meals.
- Make it a rule to never eat standing up. Eat purposefully, appreciating the tastes and textures of food.
- Take a *passegiata,* a stroll around the neighborhood with your kids or friends after dinner.

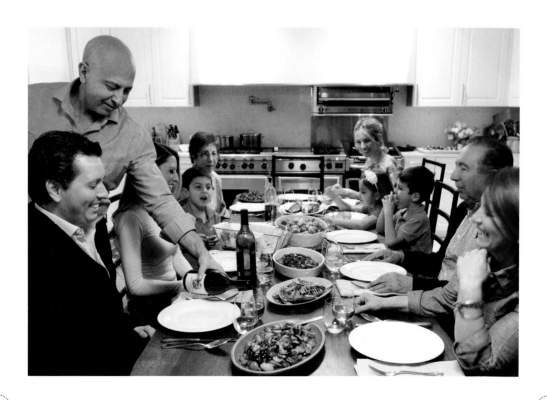

Roasted Boneless Leg of Lamb with Thyme, Garlic, and Rosemary

Leg of lamb is a relatively low-fat meat. When we compare 3 ounces of lean leg of lamb with porterhouse steak, for example, the lamb has 2 grams of saturated fat (7 grams overall) versus 10 grams (23 grams overall) for the steak—it also has half the calories.

Serve this dish with roasted potatoes or cannellini beans sautéed in garlic and sage.

SERVES 6

2 tablespoons chopped fresh thyme	1 tablespoon black pepper
2 tablespoons chopped fresh rosemary	¼ cup extra-virgin olive oil
1 tablespoon salt	4 cloves garlic, finely minced
	1 boneless leg of lamb, about 4 pounds, butterflied

1. Combine the thyme, rosemary, salt, pepper, oil, and garlic in a bowl.
2. Place the lamb on a baking pan and spread the marinade generously on both sides. You can either refrigerate it for 1 to 2 hours or proceed with cooking it.
3. Preheat the oven to 375°F.
4. Roast the lamb for 15 to 20 minutes. Increase the oven temperature to broil and broil it for another 3 to 5 minutes on each side, until an instant-read thermometer inserted into the thickest portion reaches a temperature of 145°F for medium rare.
5. To retain the succulent juices of the meat, allow the lamb to rest at room temperature for 5 minutes before slicing and serving it.

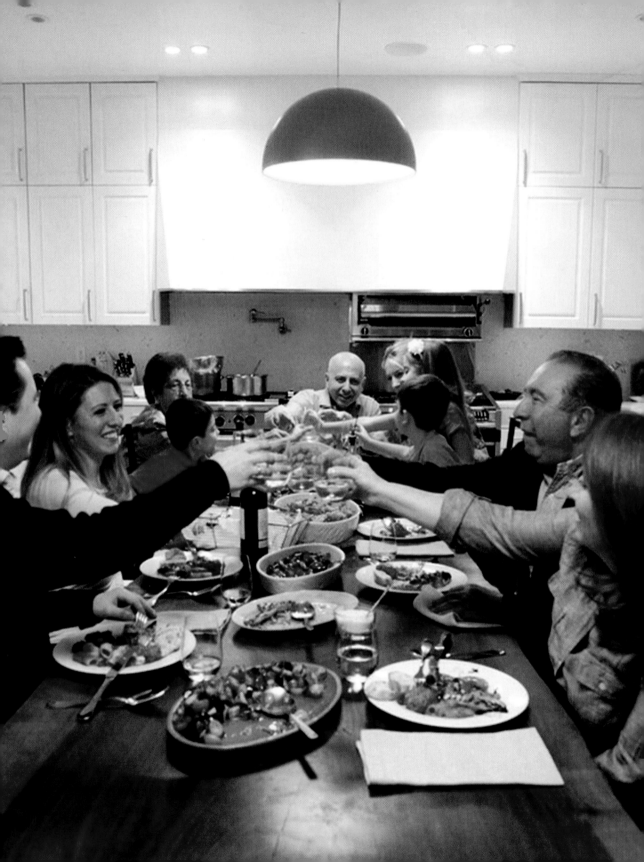

Sunday Suppers

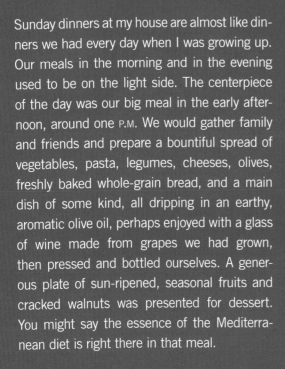

Sunday dinners at my house are almost like dinners we had every day when I was growing up. Our meals in the morning and in the evening used to be on the light side. The centerpiece of the day was our big meal in the early afternoon, around one P.M. We would gather family and friends and prepare a bountiful spread of vegetables, pasta, legumes, cheeses, olives, freshly baked whole-grain bread, and a main dish of some kind, all dripping in an earthy, aromatic olive oil, perhaps enjoyed with a glass of wine made from grapes we had grown, then pressed and bottled ourselves. A generous plate of sun-ripened, seasonal fruits and cracked walnuts was presented for dessert. You might say the essence of the Mediterranean diet is right there in that meal.

The one aspect that is unique about our Sunday meal was that we didn't (and still don't) have fish, because fish are not caught on Fridays and delivered on Saturday, so by Sunday they wouldn't have been fresh enough. Consequently, Sunday is our one day of the week when the meal revolves around a meat or poultry entrée.

Choose one suggested item from each of the categories in the following list to create your own Sunday supper. Serve it with sparkling water, flat water, and/or a glass of wine.

MEAT
Mama's Meatballs (page 269); Roasted Boneless Leg of Lamb with Thyme, Garlic, and Rosemary (page 265); Easy Baked Chicken Cutlets (page 260)

VEGETABLES *(choose two):* Carrots with Oregano and Vinegar (page 164); Roasted Broccoli with Parmigiano (page 166); Olive Oil Mashed Potatoes (page 169)

PASTA: Your choice of pasta with Quick and Easy Tomato Sauce (page 290)

SIMPLE GREEN SALAD *(choose one without a protein like chicken or fish):* Broiled Eggplant and Tomato Salad (page 140); Salad with Pecorino Cheese (page 146); Mushroom Salad (page 147)

BREAD: Italian baguette with olive oil for dipping

DESSERT: Mediterranean Dessert Platter (page 285), and if you're feeling authentic, Boiled Artichokes (page 176)

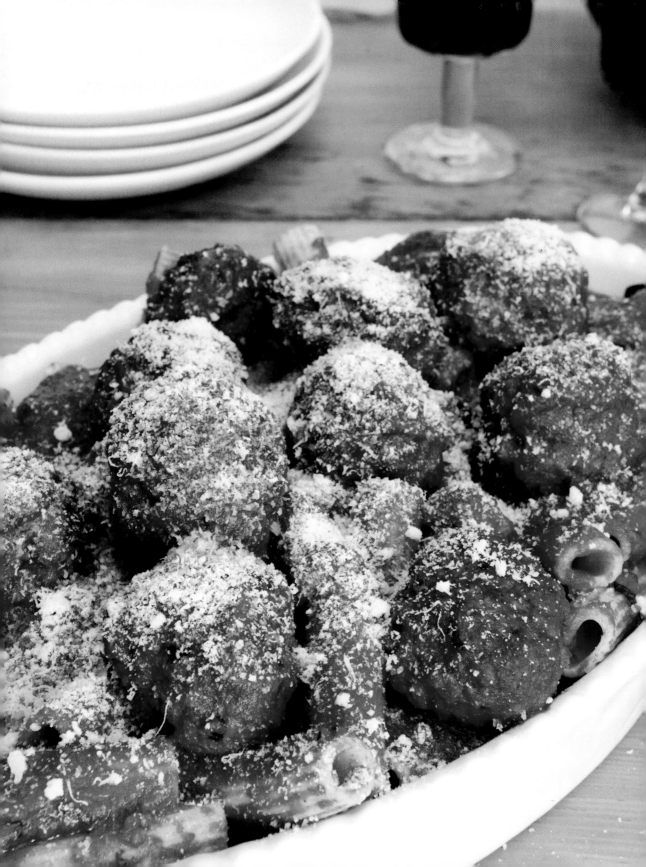

Mama's Meatballs with Pasta

Ⓚ kids

This is my mother's recipe. The secret she taught me is to allow the meatball mixture to sit for a half hour with warm water on top before sautéing the meatballs in oil. The bread crumbs will absorb the water, which imparts a soft texture.

Meatballs are one nice way to reduce meat in your diet. They tend not to be the centerpiece of a meal, but rather a hearty accessory to the pasta. They freeze very well also, so I like to make a big batch and tuck away what's left for an easy meal another day.

SERVES 8

MEATBALLS

1 pound ground pork
1 pound ground beef
1 pound ground veal
3 beaten eggs
2 cloves garlic, chopped
½ cup chopped fresh parsley

1 cup seasoned bread crumbs
⅔ cup grated Parmigiano cheese
1 tablespoon black pepper
½ tablespoon salt
½ cup canola oil
½ cup extra-virgin olive oil

PASTA

1½ to 2 quarts Quick and Easy
   Tomato Sauce (page 290)
2 tablespoons salt
2 pounds rigatoni or any short
   pasta

Grated Parmigiano cheese, for
   serving

1. To prepare the meatballs, in a large bowl, combine the meats, eggs, garlic, parsley, bread crumbs, cheese, pepper, salt, and ½ cup of water. Mix well with your hands.

2. Poke holes into the mixture with your fingers and pour another ½ cup water on top. Set this aside at room temperature for 30 minutes. This allows the mixture to absorb the moisture and makes the meatballs soft.

continued >

3. Roll the meat into balls about the size of an ice cream scoop, and place them on a large plate. You should have about 30 meatballs.

4. Put the canola and olive oils in a large pan over high heat and fry the meatballs for approximately 2 minutes on each side. Do not overcrowd the pan. Don't cook them for too long or the meatballs will lose their soft texture.

5. To complete the dish, warm the sauce in a large pot partially covered over medium heat and place the meatballs in the tomato sauce along with ½ cup of water. (This water is needed to replace what the meatballs will absorb.) Cook the sauce for 10 to 15 minutes.

6. Transfer the meatballs from the sauce to a warm serving platter. Remove the pot of sauce from the heat while you cook the pasta.

7. Bring a large pot of water to a boil over high heat. Add the salt and the rigatoni and cook it to al dente, about 9 minutes. When the pasta's almost ready, set the pot of sauce over medium heat to warm up.

8. Drain the pasta and place it directly into the pot containing the sauce; cook the pasta and sauce mixture over medium heat for about 30 seconds.

9. Place pasta portions onto individual plates, sprinkle them with cheese to taste, top each plate with 3 meatballs, and sprinkle with just a bit more cheese.

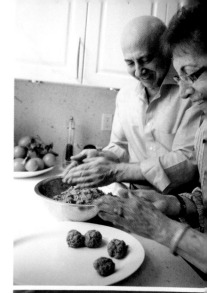

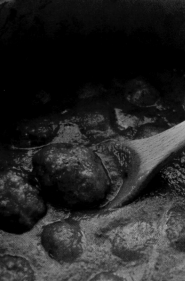

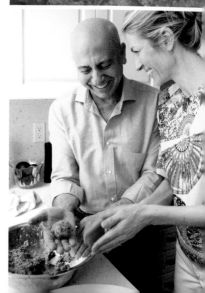

On the Grill

B babies
K kids
S seniors

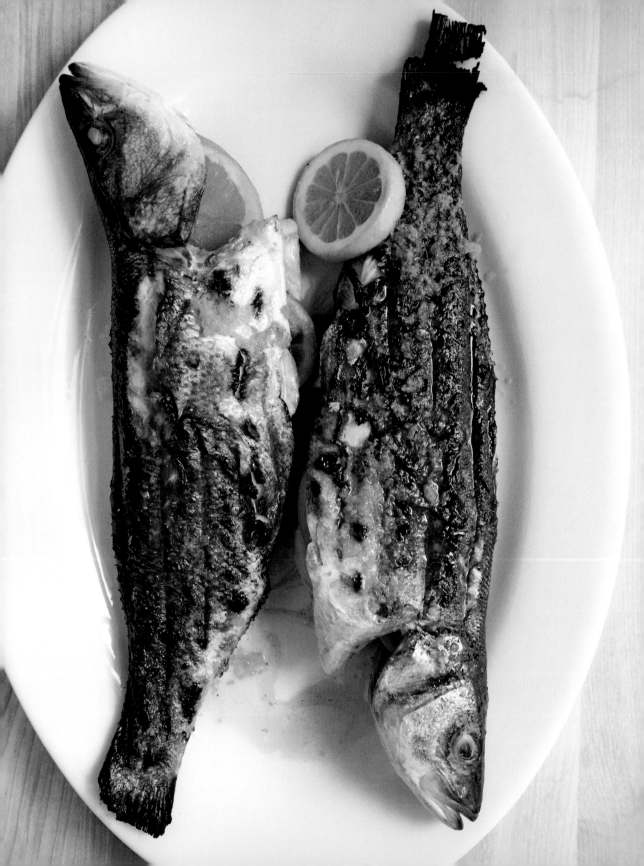

Citrus-Stuffed Branzini

⑤ seniors

This dish is one of my favorites for the grill. If a fish comes whole from the store, leave the head and tail on when you cook it, to help retain moisture. The fish is done is when the inside of the stomach is dry.

SERVES 2

2 whole branzini, cleaned
  (scaled, gutted, and fins
  removed, but head left on)
1 teaspoon salt
4 tablespoons extra-virgin olive
  oil

3 lemons
2 oranges
½ cup fresh basil leaves

1. Clean the grill or grill pan, grease it generously with olive oil (or any vegetable oil), and preheat it over medium heat.

2. Season the insides and outsides of the fish with salt, then rub them with 2 tablespoons of the olive oil.

3. Grate the zest from 1 of the lemons and 1 of the oranges; squeeze the juice from 1 of the lemons. Combine the zests and the juice and stir. Cut the remaining lemons and oranges into ¼-inch rounds. Fill the cavity of each fish with the citrus slices and the basil leaves. To the zest-and-juice mixture, add the remaining 2 tablespoons of olive oil. Stir well, then let the zest sink to the bottom.

4. Put the fish on the heated, oiled grill, using indirect medium heat, and cook with the lid closed (see Note). After grilling them for about 10 minutes on one side, turn the fish over and cook them for 7 to 10 minutes longer.

5. While the fish are still hot, spoon the oil and lemon juice mixture over them, leaving the bitter zest behind.

NOTE: I have a restaurant-style open grill in my kitchen (as seen in the photo on page 274), which is fine to leave open. However, if you have a lid on your grill, close it in this step.

Take Care When Grilling

Grilling any type of meat, even chicken or fish, until it's charred or burned can increase your exposure to cancer-causing substances, according to the American Institute for Cancer Research. (Grilling vegetables and fruits does not create carcinogens, however, so they're perfectly safe.)

If you do choose to barbecue meat, avoid burning it, and follow these tips:

Cook on a clean grill. Scrub your grill thoroughly after every use to avoid a buildup of bacteria and toxic charred residue.

Oil your grill. Grease your grill generously with olive oil or other vegetable oil before cooking. This will prevent charred material from sticking to the food and helps keep fish and chicken in one piece.

Grill fish instead of meat. Dripping fat that alights in the grill is what creates the carcinogens. Since fish contains less fat than meat and poultry, as well as requires less time on the grill to cook, carcinogen exposure is reduced.

Lower the heat. On charcoal grills, increase the distance between the food and the hot coals by spreading the coals thin or propping the grill rack on bricks. On gas grills, lower the settings.

Choose charcoal and hardwood over softwood. Barbecue briquettes and hardwood products like hickory and maple burn at lower temperatures than softwood chips like pine.

Flip meat frequently. This reduces the amount of carcinogens that accumulate. (Though let fish sit awhile so it won't stick and break apart.)

Marinate your food. Marinating not only makes grilled foods taste great, but it makes them safer because marinades tend to draw out chemical precursors of carcinogens.

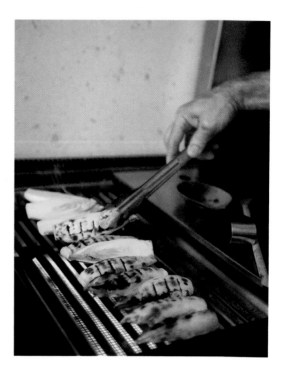

Lamb Kebabs

K kids

Serve this with Tzatziki Sauce (page 299) and a green salad, using parsley, basil, and oregano for flavoring.

SERVES 4 TO 6

2 pounds meat from leg of lamb, cut into 2-inch cubes

2 medium zucchini, cut into pieces about 2 inches long and ½ inch thick

1 large red onion, cut into wedges

1 tablespoon salt

1 tablespoon black pepper

⅓ cup extra-virgin olive oil

1 cup white wine

3 tablespoons red wine vinegar

1 tablespoon chopped fresh rosemary

1 tablespoon chopped fresh thyme

1. Combine all of the ingredients in a large bowl, cover it, and let the meat marinate for 4 to 6 hours in the refrigerator.

2. Soak 4 to 6 wooden skewers in water for 20 minutes (or use metal skewers) before assembling the kebabs. Clean the grill or grill pan, grease it generously with olive oil, and preheat it over medium heat.

3. Thread alternating pieces of lamb, zucchini, and onion onto the skewers.

4. Cook them on the grill for 2 to 3 minutes on each side.

VEGGIE-SAVING TIP: Skewer your leftover veggies and grill them!

Grilled Swordfish with Sicilian Salmoriglio

Salmoriglio refers to the type of marinade used in this recipe, a blend of the ingredients below. It's a southern Italian condiment with many variations.

SERVES 4 TO 6

1 teaspoon salt

Juice of 1 lemon

1 tablespoon chopped fresh oregano, or ½ tablespoon dried

2 tablespoons chopped fresh parsley

¼ cup extra-virgin olive oil

1 teaspoon black pepper

2 pounds swordfish, cut into ½-inch slices

1. Clean the grill or grill pan, grease it generously with olive oil, and preheat it over medium heat.

2. To make the salmoriglio, in a medium bowl, beat the salt and the lemon juice with a fork until the salt has dissolved. Stir in the oregano and parsley and slowly add the oil, drop by drop, while beating with a fork; the oil and lemon must emulsify. Add the pepper and set the sauce aside.

3. Grill the swordfish for 2 minutes on one side and 30 minutes on the other side.

4. Place the fish on a warm serving platter and drizzle on the salmoriglio while the fish is still hot. Serve warm.

Grilled Langoustines

I recently made this dish for a group of colleagues, many of whom were not familiar with langoustines—narrow crustaceans about 6 inches long that look like a cross between a lobster and a shrimp, with similar textured meat that is sweeter than crabmeat. They said they'd never tasted anything so sweet. One diner has been seeking them out at Cipriani ever since, as he says they're one of his favorite dishes. Langoustines are always sold frozen in the United States, so you can always ask your fishmonger to get them for you, and then defrost them at home before you cook them. A chopped radicchio salad with lemon and olive oil dressing goes very nicely with them.

SERVES 4

16 langoustines
Extra-virgin olive oil

½ teaspoon salt
1 lemon, cut into 4 wedges

1. Clean the grill or grill pan, grease it generously with olive oil, and preheat it over medium heat.
2. Cut the langoustines in half lengthwise. Brush the inner halves with olive oil and sprinkle them with the salt.
3. Place them on the hot grill, shell side down, and grill for 3 to 4 minutes, until the meat is translucent, similar to cooked shrimp.
4. Turn the langoustines meat side down for 10 seconds and then transfer them to a warm serving platter. Drizzle them with a little more oil and serve them with lemon wedges.

Salmon Kebabs

K kids **S** seniors

SERVES 8

DRESSING

Juice of 4 lemons

½ teaspoon white wine vinegar

¼ cup chopped fresh parsley

¼ cup chopped fresh cilantro

5 cloves garlic, finely chopped

1 teaspoon ground cumin

½ teaspoon cayenne

2 tablespoons paprika

⅔ cup extra-virgin olive oil

KEBABS

2 pounds skinless salmon, cut
    into 1½-inch cubes

2 medium eggplants, cut into
    ½-inch chunks

2 medium zucchinis, cut into
    ½-inch chunks

1 large Vidalia or other sweet
    onion, cut into 1-inch wedges

¼ cup extra-virgin olive oil

Salt and black pepper

1 lemon, cut into 6 wedges

1. Soak 10 wooden skewers in water for 20 minutes (or use metal skewers) before assembling the kebabs. Clean the grill or grill pan, generously grease it with olive oil, and preheat it over medium heat.

2. To make the dressing, in a mixing bowl, combine the lemon juice, vinegar, parsley, cilantro, garlic, cumin, cayenne, and paprika; pour the oil in slowly in a thin stream while whisking.

3. Thread the salmon and vegetables, in alternation, onto the skewers. Use the oil to brush both the salmon and vegetables on all sides; this is important to keep the kebabs from sticking to the grill. Season them with salt and pepper.

4. Grill the kebabs for approximately 8 minutes, turning them four times for even cooking. Place them all on a large serving platter immediately, drizzling them with the dressing, and providing wedges of lemon on the side.

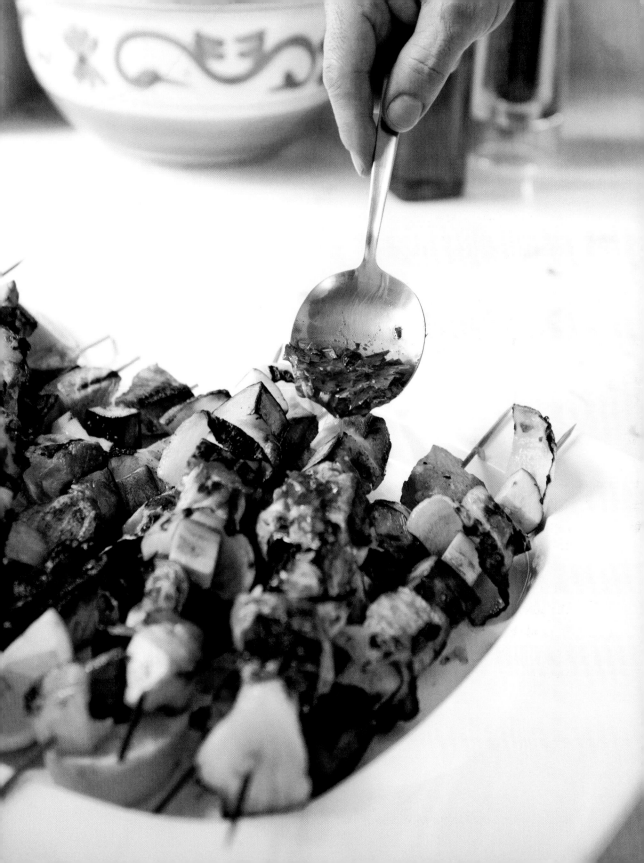

Grilled Endive with Balsamic

SERVES 6

8 Belgian endives, cut in half
   lengthwise
5 tablespoons extra-virgin olive
   oil
½ teaspoon salt

2 tablespoons balsamic
   reduction (see the footnote on
   page 77)
2 tablespoons toasted pine nuts

1. Clean the grill or grill pan, generously grease it with olive oil, and preheat it over medium heat.

2. Lightly coat the endives with 3 tablespoons of the olive oil.

3. Place the endives onto the grill and cook them for 2 to 4 minutes on each side.

4. Place the endives onto a serving platter, sprinkle them with salt, drizzle them with the remaining 2 tablespoons of oil and the balsamic reduction, and sprinkle them with pine nuts.

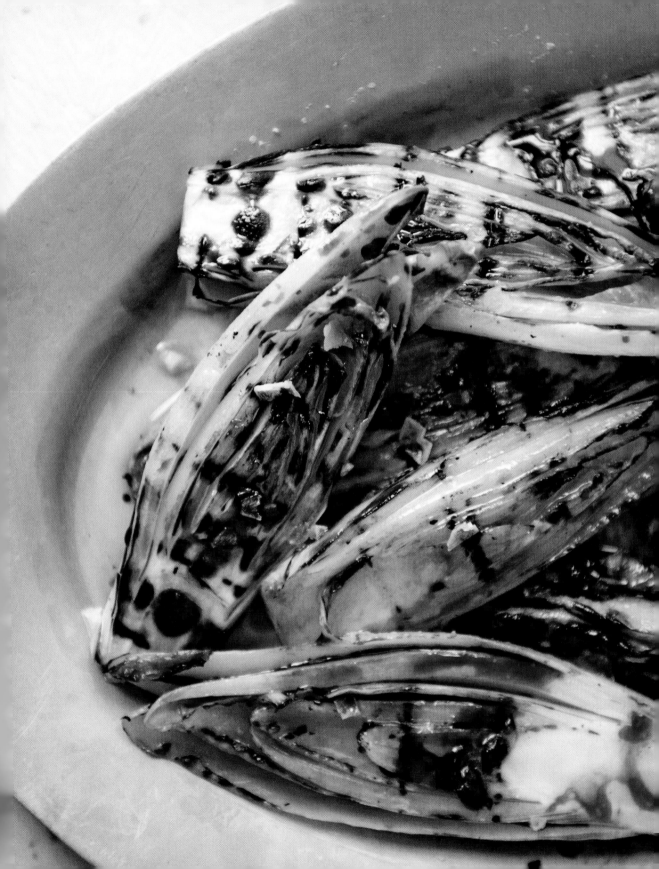

Grilled Chicken Cutlets

SERVES 4

4 chicken cutlets, evenly
   pounded to ½ inch thick
1 teaspoon salt
1 teaspoon black pepper

6 cloves garlic, sliced
1 tablespoon chopped fresh
   rosemary
¼ cup extra-virgin olive oil

1. Place the cutlets, salt, pepper, garlic, rosemary, and olive oil in a resealable plastic bag and let them marinate in the refrigerator for 2 to 3 hours.

2. Clean the grill or grill pan, grease it generously with olive oil, and preheat it over medium heat.

3. Shake off the garlic and grill the cutlets for 2 to 3 minutes on each side.

Desserts

🅑 babies

🅚 kids

🅢 seniors

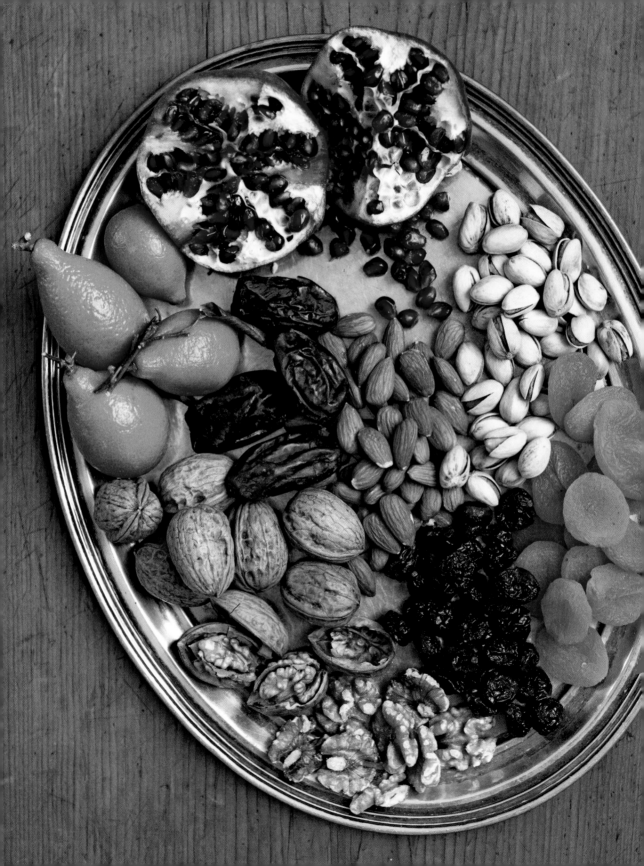

Mediterranean Dessert Platter

I don't have a lot of dessert recipes in my book, because southern Italians didn't often have a prepared dessert after a meal in the 1950s and '60s. Instead, we would have a piece of fresh fruit, or sometimes boiled artichokes (see page 176). This dessert platter is what was typically set before us after a meal. Nuts in the shell always taste better, and they're fun to crack open, especially when children are around. It takes time, which allows people to linger at the kitchen table and make small talk. This is what eating Sicilian is all about.

Apricots

Figs

Dates

In-season fresh fruit

Walnuts

Other nuts to your liking, such as almonds, cashews, and pistachios

Place a colorful mixture of the above on a large platter and set it in the middle of the table for sharing. Include a nutcracker if you serve any nuts in their shells.

Fresh Fennel Dessert

When it's in season, I serve fennel as a refreshing—perhaps unexpected—dessert.

1 fennel bulb

1. Wash the fennel and remove the fronds and hard outer husk.
2. Slice the fennel bulb into four pieces, and place them on a dish. Best enjoyed cold.

Mixed Nut Crumble

K kids **S** seniors

We keep this in the house all the time. It serves as a sweet and healthy snack or dessert—without any added sugar!

SERVES 6 TO 8

5 pitted dates (make sure they're soft; if they're hard, they're stale)
1 cup pumpkin seeds
1 cup sunflower seeds

1 cup old-fashioned rolled oats
½ cup sunflower seed butter or peanut butter
¼ cup honey
1 cup dried cranberries

1. Preheat the oven to 400°F.

2. Put the pitted dates in a blender and blend until they turn into a small ball.

3. Spread the pumpkin seeds, sunflower seeds, and oats onto a baking pan, toast them in the oven for 10 minutes, and allow them to cool to room temperature.

4. Mix the sunflower seed butter and honey in a small pan over low heat. Cook and stir for 4 minutes until the mixture loosens.

5. In a large bowl, combine the toasted seeds and oats, the cranberries, blended dates, and sunflower seed butter mixture and stir until everything is well combined.

6. Line an 8 × 8-inch baking dish with a sheet of plastic wrap, allowing the plastic to overlap the rimmed edges. Mold the crumble mixture into the dish using your hands and pressing firmly.

7. Allow the crumble to harden for 1 hour in the freezer or for a few hours in the refrigerator.

8. Remove it from the dish by pulling on the plastic wrap and then peel off the plastic. Place the crumble on a cutting board and cut it into 1- to 2-inch squares. Store it in an airtight container for up to 2 weeks.

Dressings and Sauces

Ⓑ babies
Ⓚ kids
Ⓢ seniors

Fresh Plum Tomato Sauce

This recipe yields a sauce with a concentrated flavor that beats anything from a jar! This takes a bit of work, but it is worth the time invested, and it freezes well if you want to make a large batch to store. Be sure to use a food mill (a utensil for mashing and sieving soft foods), as it's important to remove the tomato seeds and peels to achieve the best flavor.

SERVES 4 TO 6
(ENOUGH SAUCE FOR 1½ TO 2 POUNDS OF PASTA)

4 pounds plum tomatoes,
  washed and cut into quarters
1 teaspoon salt
6 tablespoons extra-virgin
  olive oil

4 cloves garlic, crushed
½ teaspoon red pepper flakes
1 tablespoon tomato paste
1 teaspoon sugar
10 fresh basil leaves, chopped

1. Place the tomatoes and salt in a large pot over high heat, bring it to a boil, then lower the heat to simmer the sauce, partially covered, for 30 minutes.

2. Place a food mill over a pot and process the tomatoes through it. This will yield a puree in the pot, with the seeds and tomato skins left behind in the food mill bowl.

3. Bring the puree to a boil, then lower the heat to a simmer, leaving the pot uncovered. Cook for 30 minutes, stirring occasionally. This will concentrate the sauce.

4. Put the oil in a large pan over medium heat, and add the garlic, red pepper flakes, and tomato paste. Sauté for 30 seconds, then add the tomato puree, sugar, and basil. Cook for 5 minutes, and you're ready to put this sauce on any pasta.

> **VEGGIE-SAVING TIP:** If your tomatoes are starting to turn, it's time to make tomato sauce!

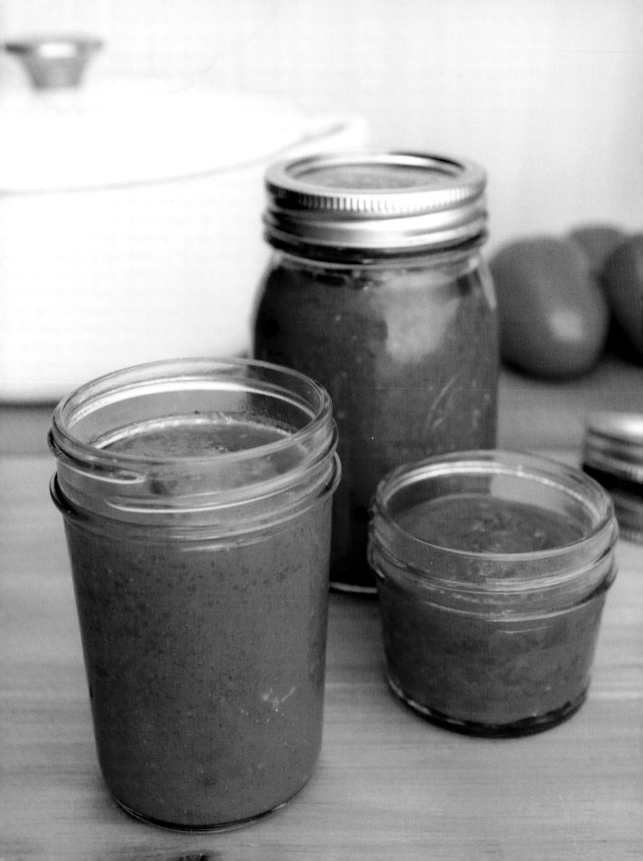

Quick and Easy Tomato Sauce

K kids

This is my wife's new favorite tomato sauce—she loves the taste. Its success depends entirely on the type of tomatoes you use (as I've mentioned, I highly recommend DOP San Marzano tomatoes) and on blending the garlic well into the sauce.

SERVES 4 (ENOUGH SAUCE FOR 1 POUND OF PASTA)

1 (28-ounce) can San Marzano
   whole peeled plum tomatoes
¼ cup extra-virgin olive oil
½ teaspoon red pepper flakes
1 tablespoon tomato paste

6 cloves garlic, sliced
3 tablespoons chopped fresh
   basil
1 teaspoon salt
1 teaspoon sugar

1. Put the tomatoes into a bowl and coarsely squish them with your hands, reserving the juice.

2. Put the oil in a large pan over medium heat and add the red pepper flakes, tomato paste, and garlic. Sauté the garlic for 1 minute and add the tomatoes with their juices, 2 tablespoons of the chopped basil, the salt, and the sugar.

3. Bring the mixture to a boil, lower the heat, cover the pan, and simmer for 10 to 15 minutes, stirring occasionally.

4. Use an immersion blender to puree the sauce. The cooked garlic blends into the sauce and gives it a wonderful flavor.

5. Add the last tablespoon of basil when you mix the sauce with the pasta.

Oil and Vinegar Salad Dressing

If you have never made your own salad dressing before, you will be amazed at how flavorful it can be without the salt and sugar that dominate store-bought dressing! Some people like the tart flavor of red and white wine vinegar, and some don't. For those who don't, balsamic salad dressing preparations are sweeter and not as pungent.

For salad dressings where you need to blend oil into nonoily ingredients, vigorous side-to-side whisking as you slowly pour the oil in provides the speed and sheer force to break the oil into tinier droplets, allowing them to stay suspended in lemon juice or vinegar for as long as possible. Because emulsification doesn't last, I recommend that you prepare these salad dressings just before you're going to dress the salads (or at a minimum, use them within twenty-four hours). They'll taste best fresh, and if stored, they'll congeal and lose their well-blended consistency.

SERVES 4

RED OR WHITE WINE
3 to 4 tablespoons red or white wine vinegar
Salt and pepper to taste
¼ cup extra-virgin olive oil

BALSAMIC
3 to 4 tablespoons balsamic vinegar
½ teaspoon salt
½ teaspoon black pepper
¼ teaspoon dried oregano
¼ cup extra-virgin olive oil

Choose your desired vinaigrette and combine the vinegar and seasonings in a small bowl. While whisking, pour the oil into the vinegar mixture slowly, until the dressing emulsifies. Drizzle the dressing over any salad.

Low-Fat Sicilian Caesar Dressing

While most Caesar salad dressings are prepared with raw eggs, this one doesn't call for them, saving you the calories, cholesterol, and food poisoning risk, but still keeping that wonderful Caesar taste. This dressing is excellent on kale salad, especially with 1 to 2 tablespoons of shaved Parmigiano on top. Prepare the salad in advance and refrigerate it so that you can serve it chilled, then make the dressing just before you're ready to toss it.

SERVES 4 TO 6

1 clove garlic, finely minced
2 tablespoons balsamic vinegar
1 tablespoon Dijon mustard
4 anchovy fillets, chopped
Pinch of salt

2 tablespoons grated Parmigiano cheese
1 teaspoon Worcestershire sauce
6 tablespoons extra-virgin olive oil

1. Combine all the ingredients except the olive oil in a blender and puree until well mixed, 15 to 20 seconds.
2. Pour the contents into a bowl. While whisking, pour in the olive oil slowly. Drizzle the dressing over any salad.

Cream of Avocado

This sauce goes wonderfully with all kinds of seafood, including grilled. It can be used as a topping, a dipping sauce, or a bed for any seafood. For instance, try salmon steaks seasoned with salt and drizzled with olive oil on a bed of avocado cream. It's delicious.

Use ripe avocados, because they're more flavorful and will take on the creamy consistency that you want. Look for avocados that are medium green and slightly tender when squeezed (hard or mushy are either too young or too old, respectively).

SERVES 4

1 red onion, chopped
3 tablespoons extra-virgin olive
   oil
½ red chile pepper

Salt
Flesh of 2 medium-size ripe
   avocados

1. Combine the red onion, olive oil, red pepper, and salt in a blender and puree.
2. Add the avocado and blend until the mixture is smooth, creamy, and velvety.

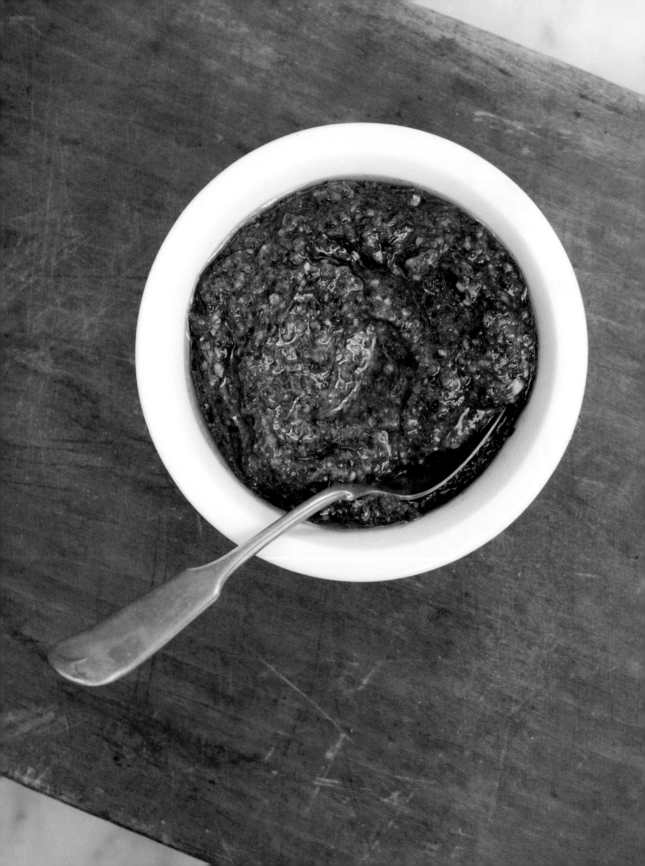

Pesto Sauce, Four Ways

Different regions of Italy have different types of pesto, depending on what's grown locally. In Sicily, almonds are abundant, so the typical pesto is almond-based rather than pignoli. Because cherry tomatoes are also so plentiful, and sweet, we use those in our traditional pesto as well. Broccoli rabe is also commonly grown in Sicily, so broccoli rabe pesto is often made. Get off the beaten path of pine-nut pesto, and try new versions of this wonderful pasta sauce.

Serve it with pasta, with bread, on top of meat, or alongside vegetables.

Traditional

Fresh basil has antioxidant, antimicrobial, and anti-inflammatory properties. Because it oxidizes quickly and turns black, the spinach is nice to add to the recipe—it keeps the pesto green. Serve this pesto with spaghetti or any short pasta.

SERVES 4
(ENOUGH SAUCE FOR 1 POUND OF PASTA)

1 handful of nuts (such as pignoli, almonds, or walnuts)

1 cup fresh baby spinach, washed and dried

2 cups fresh basil leaves, washed and dried

Pinch of salt, optional

1 clove garlic

½ cup extra-virgin olive oil

¼ cup grated Parmigiano cheese

1. Toast the nuts in a dry sauté pan over medium heat for no more than 1 to 2 minutes. Watch them carefully, as they burn quickly.

2. Put the spinach, basil, and nuts in a blender, along with the salt (if using) and garlic. Start blending as you slowly drizzle in the olive oil. When the oil has been incorporated, add the cheese and blend for another 10 to 15 seconds. I often reserve 3 to 4 tablespoons of pasta cooking water to add if I feel the consistency of the pesto is too thick.

3. You may want to drizzle on a little extra olive oil and sprinkle the pasta with cheese before serving, for added flavor.

Trapanese

This pesto recipe comes from the Sicilian town of Trapani. Serve it with short pasta like penne fusilli or caserecce.

SERVES 4 (ENOUGH SAUCE FOR 1 POUND OF PASTA)

1 handful almonds
1 clove garlic, chopped
2½ cups fresh basil leaves
1 cup cherry tomatoes

½ cup extra-virgin olive oil, plus
  more as needed
½ cup grated Parmigiano cheese
Salt and black pepper

1. Toast the almonds in a dry sauté pan over medium heat for no more than 1 to 2 minutes. Watch them carefully, as they burn quickly.

2. Place the garlic and toasted almonds into a blender and blend for 10 to 15 seconds.

3. Add the basil and tomatoes and blend for another 20 to 30 seconds, while slowly adding the olive oil. Blend well enough that you don't see the tomato skins (if you can see them, the texture will be very unpleasant to the palate).

4. Add the Parmigiano and a pinch of salt and pepper, and blend for another 10 to 20 seconds.

5. If the pesto is a little thick, you may add a few tablespoons of the pasta cooking water or olive oil to loosen it up.

Broccoli Rabe

My favorite way to serve this pesto sauce is mixed into spaghetti, topped with a drizzle of olive oil, some of the sautéed broccoli rabe florets, and a sprinkle of Parmigiano.

SERVES 4 (ENOUGH SAUCE FOR 1 POUND OF PASTA)

2 bunches broccoli rabe

1 tablespoon plus ¼ teaspoon salt

9 tablespoons extra-virgin olive oil

4 cloves garlic, sliced

Pinch of red pepper flakes

4 anchovy fillets, chopped

¼ cup grated Parmigiano cheese

1. Wash and trim the broccoli rabe, reserving the top 2 to 3 inches of the florets. Set aside. Roughly chop the remaining upper stems and leaves.

2. Bring a pot filled with about 1 quart of water to a boil over high heat. Add 1 tablespoon of the salt and the broccoli rabe stems and leaves. Boil for 2 to 3 minutes.

3. Reserve 1 cup of the cooking water and drain the broccoli rabe stems and leaves. Place them, along with ½ cup of the reserved cooking water, in a blender.

4. Put 3 tablespoons of the olive oil in a large pan over medium heat and add half of the sliced garlic, the red pepper flakes, and the anchovies. Cook until the garlic is golden and the anchovies have melted into the oil.

5. Add the oil mixture and the broccoli rabe stems and leaves to the blender, along with the cheese and 4 tablespoons of the oil. Blend well until the mixture liquefies into a sauce, adding more of the reserved cooking water from the broccoli rabe if necessary, until you reach the consistency of a pureed tomato sauce. Pour it into a large serving bowl.

6. In the same pan that contained the garlic and anchovies, heat the remaining 2 tablespoons of oil over medium heat and sauté the remaining sliced garlic.

7. When the garlic turns golden, add the broccoli rabe florets and the remaining ¼ teaspoon of salt. The wet-washed broccoli rabe should already have enough water; if not, add 2 tablespoons of water and cook for 3 minutes on low to medium heat, tossing occasionally. Top the pasta with the broccoli rabe florets before serving.

Kale and Basil

Enjoy this pesto with spaghetti, penne, or ziti.

SERVES 4 (ENOUGH SAUCE FOR 1 POUND OF PASTA)

¼ cup walnut halves

1 clove garlic, chopped

½ teaspoon salt

½ teaspoon black pepper

2½ cups kale leaves, any type, stems removed and leaves roughly cut into 1-inch strips

2 cups fresh basil leaves

½ cup extra-virgin olive oil

½ cup grated Parmigiano cheese

1. Toast the walnuts in a dry sauté pan over medium heat for 3 to 4 minutes, tossing frequently to avoid burning.

2. To a blender add the garlic, salt, pepper, and walnuts; blend for 10 to 20 seconds.

3. Add the kale and basil, and slowly drizzle in half of the olive oil, blending until the contents are well incorporated, 40 to 60 seconds.

4. Add the cheese and the remaining oil, and blend for another 20 to 30 seconds.

5. Add a bit of the pasta cooking water, up to ¼ cup, until the pesto reaches your desired consistency. I prefer the thickness of a tomato sauce.

> TIP: A nice advantage of pesto is that it stores easily in the freezer, so it makes very convenient meals. If you're making a batch to freeze, prepare it without the cheese. Make a little extra and freeze it in individual plastic tubs. To thaw, all you have to do is put the frozen pesto in a pot on the stove, add 2 to 4 tablespoons of water, and heat it on a low flame until it thaws and warms. Once it softens, stir in the desired amount of cheese.

Tzatziki Sauce

 kids

Tzatziki is a classic, chilled yogurt-based Mediterranean sauce. It's a very refreshing accompaniment to so many things—all kinds of fish and meat—especially anything off the grill. It can also be used as a dip for veggies or pita bread or kebabs, spread onto sandwiches, mixed in with mashed potatoes, and even tossed into salad as a dressing. Experiment and enjoy!

SERVES 4

1 cup plain Greek yogurt

¼ cup chopped fresh dill

½ teaspoon salt

½ cup shredded seeded cucumber

Juice of ½ lemon

1 clove garlic, finely chopped

Mix all of the ingredients in a bowl. Tzatziki can be stored for up to 3 days in the refrigerator.

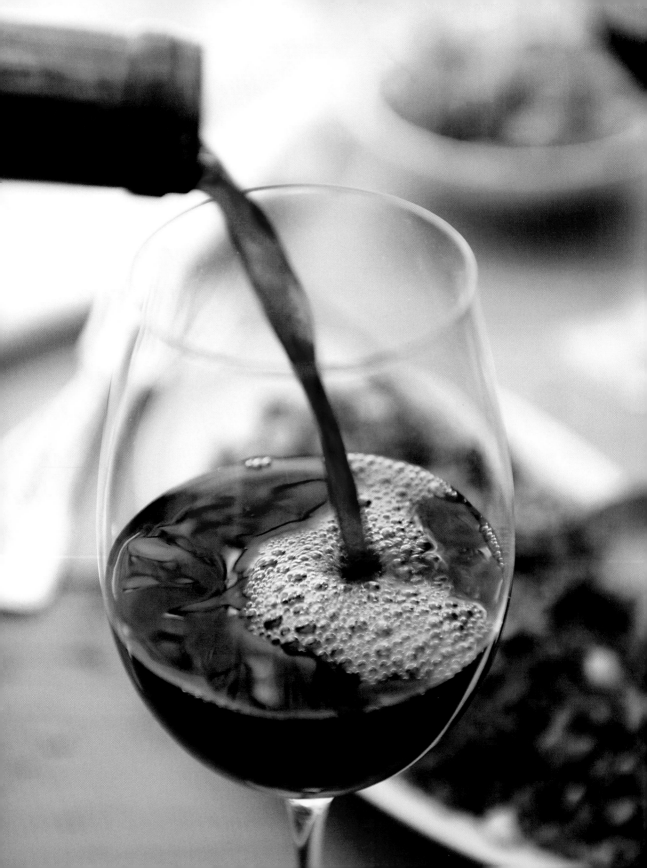

GRAZIE

There are many I am deeply indebted to for helping bring this book to life. First and foremost, my wife, Svetlana, who has been an inspiration to all I have accomplished in the time that I have known her. Her love and dedication to the family have 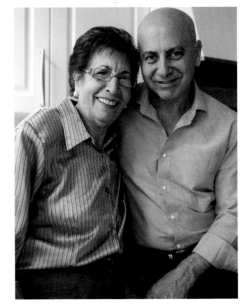 made it possible for me to do those things that I love so much. My mother, Sara, who has instilled in me the passion for food, and the love for people. And my children, Alessandra, Salvatore, and Nicholas, who add vitality to my life each and every day, and who inspired me to write this book about the Mediterranean family table.

To my medical writer, Laurie Anne Vandermolen, without whom this book would not have been possible, I sincerely thank you for your dedication, perseverance, loyalty, and attention to getting it all right. Your countless hours of research, writing, rewriting, and more rewriting were appreciated beyond measure.

To my agent extraordinaire, Laura Dail, thank you for believing in this book, for launching it into being, for propelling it to the finish line, and for the vision to make it more than we dreamed it could be. Your enthusiastic support has been appreciated and responsible for many of my literary endeavors coming to fruition.

I also wish to pay tribute to the outstanding team at HarperCollins. Thank you to editor Rebecca Hunt for helping us shape the book initially. To Cara Bedick, our talented editor with the William Morrow group, I thank you for your invaluable advice, suggestions, insight, careful editing, and above all patience while we slow-cooked this into existence.

I am also grateful to Steve Hochberg, for supporting this venture—at times an adventure—from start to finish.

To Anwesha Basu and Dianna Garcia, thank you for your important work in getting the message out. Your efforts may add years to the lives of those you reach and inspire.

To my designer, Suet Chong, thank you for the visual conception and composition that turned the text of my chapters and recipes into a stunning, full-color cookbook, along with photographer Liz Clayman and stylist Rebekah Peppler.

I also wish to express my utmost gratitude to the many chefs from Italy who provided their recipes to me, who allowed me into their kitchens and shared with me not only their preparations but also their affection. I offer special thanks to Massimo Carbone, executive chef from Brio Restaurant in New York, who always makes my lunch or dinner exciting with the many things that I like. And last but certainly not least, I offer my sincere appreciation for the support of my dear friends Michael Dowling, Mark Solazzo, Howard Gold, John Odermat, Piere Guerci, Guiseppi Cipriani, and William Hyman, whom I am always happy to see and cook for in my house and for whom I will have a seat at my table for the rest of my life.

—A.A.

I wish to thank Angelo for collaborating on yet another meaningful project that may affect the lives of so many for the better. His wisdom, charisma, authenticity, and amazing recipes truly gave this book its heart. (My family also thanks him for the cook I have become!) I would also like to express my appreciation to all those who supported us and were responsible for the book coming to be—Laura Dail, who green-lighted it and expertly guided us; Steve Hochberg, whose alliance was the water keeping the boat afloat; Rebecca Hunt, for pointing us in the right direction; Cara Bedick, for her overall vision, incisive ideas, and ever-thoughtful, gracious, and dependable assistance; and everyone else at HarperCollins whose great work helped develop and refine our illustrations and manuscript. Most important, I wish to acknowledge those at my own family table, who have been so very patient while this book got written and who bring me so much love and joy. To Bob, Peter, Julia, and Graham especially, I heart you to infinity and beyond, and even more than that.

—L.A.V.

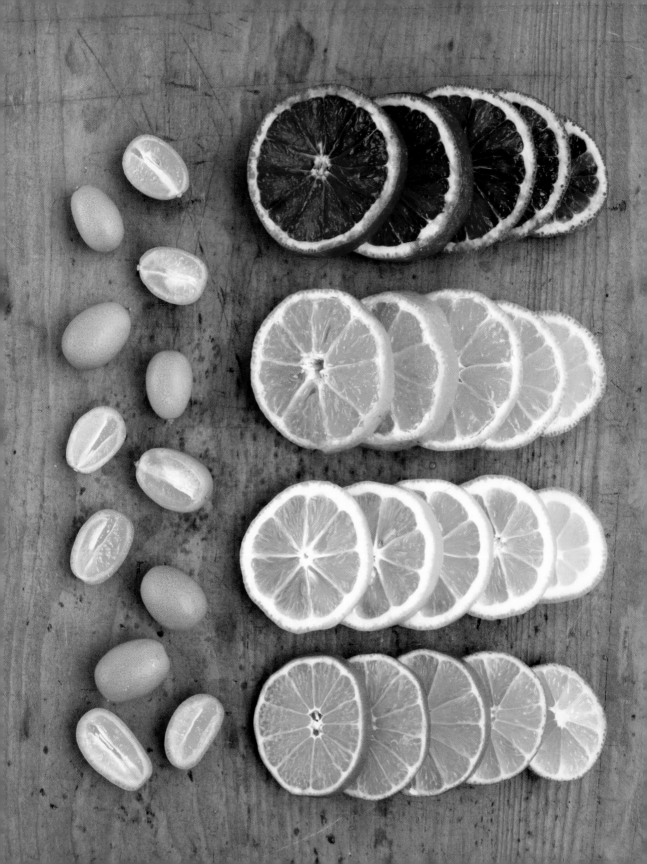

APPENDIX

SOURCES FOR NUTRIENTS

NUTRIENT	FOOD SOURCE	NOTES
Protein[X]	Dairy products Eggs Meat Seafood Nuts Seeds Legumes Cauliflower Broccoli rabe	PREGNANCY Protein is crucial for the baby's growth, especially during the second and third trimesters. THE GROWING YEARS Adequate protein is critical to reach full growth potential. Maximize vegetable proteins over animal proteins.
Healthy fats[X]	MAXIMIZE: **Monounsaturated fat** (found in olive oil, canola oil, avocados, olives) **The omega-3 polyunsaturated fat, linolenic acid** (found in walnuts and other nuts, flax) **The omega-3 polyunsaturated fats EPA and DHA** (found in oily fish like salmon, mackerel, sardines, anchovies)	DHA is especially important during pregnancy and breastfeeding for developing, growing babies. Minimize saturated fats (found in red meat, butter, and whole-fat dairy products).

[X] Important for pregnancy

NUTRIENT	FOOD SOURCE	NOTES
Healthy fats[X] *(continued)*	HEALTHY BUT DON'T OVERDO IT: **The omega-6 polyunsaturated fat, linoleic acid** (found in soybeans, soybean oil, and oils like corn, sunflower, and safflower)	Completely avoid trans fats (found in fried foods and many commercially processed foods like snacks, cookies, frozen treats, and bottled dressings).
Healthy carbohydrates	Fruits Vegetables Whole-grain products like bread, oats (steel-cut or rolled/old-fashioned), cereals, and crackers Durum semolina pasta	On labels, make sure it says "whole" before wheat (like 100% whole wheat flour and 100% whole-grain) and that it's the first item on the ingredients list. "Multigrain," "wheat flour," "enriched," or "stone-ground wheat" flour may still be refined white flour. Avoid refined carbs (like egg noodles, white bread, instant grains, and white rice).
Fluid	Water	Sugar decreases absorption. Children and seniors are more prone to dehydration.
Fiber*	Fruits—especially apples and pears (with peels), raspberries, bananas, oranges, strawberries, dried fruits Vegetables—especially broccoli, broccoli rabe, peas, corn, eggplant (with skin on), fennel Legumes Whole-grain products like oats, barley Nuts	Will help seniors diminish constipation.
Biotin[X]	Eggs Salmon Avocados Cauliflower Raspberries	Type of B vitamin.

[X] Important for pregnancy
* Often found to be deficient in children

NUTRIENT	FOOD SOURCE	NOTES
Choline[X]	Eggs Pork tenderloin Cod Salmon Chicken Broccoli Cauliflower	Helps prevent neural tube defects in developing fetuses.
Calcium[~*◊X±]	Milk and other dairy products Canned salmon or sardines Broccoli Broccoli rabe Collard greens Kale Turnips Soy products	Adequate amounts are vital during the growing years to achieve growth potential and develop strong bones. Vitamin D and vitamin C increase absorption. Caffeine interferes with absorption. Absorption declines with age. Important to meet requirements in pregnancy, but no need to supplement.
Copper	Radicchio Kiwi Leeks Fennel Beets Shellfish Whole grains Beans Nuts	An essential trace mineral, it works with iron to help the body form red blood cells and helps keep the blood vessels, nerves, immune system, and bones healthy.
Folate (and the man-made form, folic acid)[X±]	Cooked legumes (like black-eyed peas, great northern beans) Cooked spinach Dark green leafy vegetables Broccoli Broccoli rabe	Lowers homocysteine levels, which are a risk factor for heart disease. For pregnant women, helps prevent certain birth defects.

~ Important for babies   * Often found to be deficient in children

± Often found to be deficient in teens   ◊ Often found to be deficient in the elderly

X Important for pregnancy

NUTRIENT	FOOD SOURCE	NOTES
Folate (and the man-made form, folic acid)$^{X\pm}$ *(continued)*	Asparagus Enriched pasta Cantaloupe Eggs Leeks Zucchini Fennel Beets Fruits Nuts Dairy products Fortified cereals (folic acid)	Lowers homocysteine levels, which are a risk factor for heart disease. For pregnant women, helps prevent certain birth defects.
Iodine	Iodized salt Seafood Dairy products Many processed foods	A trace mineral found naturally in the body, it's needed for metabolism and normal thyroid function. Deficiency occurs more in women than in men, and is more common in pregnant women and older children.
Iron$^{*\sim\pm}$	Meat Legumes Fortified cereals Dried fruits Liver Leafy green vegetables Broccoli rabe Peas Fish Poultry Beets Blackstrap molasses	Proteins and vitamin C (especially if consumed in the same meal) increase absorption. Too much fiber at one time and large single doses decrease absorption (several smaller doses are better). Stored more readily in the elderly; too much contributes to oxidation; vitamin C increases uptake and acts as antioxidant. Iron deficiency is more common in teenage girls than in boys.

$\sim$ Important for babies   * Often found to be deficient in children

$\pm$ Often found to be deficient in teens ^{X} Important for pregnancy

NUTRIENT	FOOD SOURCE	NOTES
Lutein	Leafy green vegetables like spinach and kale Broccoli Radicchio Grapes Oranges Egg yolks	May help protect against age-related macular degeneration of the eyes.
Lycopene	Tomatoes, especially cooked Watermelon	Potent antioxidant found in red fruits and vegetables.
Lysine	Red meat Nuts Legumes, especially soybeans	Helps the body absorb calcium; important for bone and connective tissue growth.
Magnesium$^\lozenge$	Legumes Nuts Seeds Fish Whole grains Molasses Chocolate	Important for muscle, nerve, and bone health.
Phosphorus	Milk Dairy products Meat Fish Eggs Whole grains Legumes Fennel Beets	Plays an important role in bone and teeth formation and carbohydrate and fat metabolism, and is needed for the body to make protein for growth and repair of cells and tissues. Phosphorus also helps the body make ATP, a molecule the body uses to store energy. Carbonated beverages decrease absorption.
Phytoestrogens	Oilseeds like flaxseed and sesame seeds Soy products Legumes	Especially important for menopausal women.

$\lozenge$ Often found to be deficient in the elderly

NUTRIENT	FOOD SOURCE	NOTES
Phytoestrogens *(continued)*	Whole grains like oats, cracked wheat, barley Meat products Fruits like apples, pomegranates Vegetables like carrots, yams, alfalfa, fennel Coffee	Especially important for menopausal women.
Potassium◊	Fruits like bananas, oranges, cantaloupe, raisins, kiwis Legumes like white beans Vegetables like winter squash, spinach, sweet and white potatoes (skins on), broccoli, eggplant (skin on) Whole grains Fresh meats Yogurt Fish Zucchini Fennel Beets Tomato paste	Helps balance sodium in the diet.
Selenium	Nuts Canned tuna Bell peppers	Antioxidant properties.
Vitamin A~	Sweet potato Carrots Green leafy vegetables Broccoli rabe Ricotta cheese Cantaloupe Apricots Pickled herring Milk Eggs Red bell peppers Mangoes	Helps form and maintain healthy skin, teeth, bones, and skin. Promotes good vision. May be needed for reproduction and breastfeeding. Can be too high in the elderly.

~ Important for babies ◊ Often found to be deficient in the elderly

NUTRIENT	FOOD SOURCE	NOTES
Vitamin B_6	Sunflower seeds Pistachio nuts Fish Meats like turkey, chicken, lean pork Dried fruits (especially prunes) Bananas Avocados Spinach Chickpeas Eggplant Beets Zucchini Leeks	Plays an important role in energy, fat, and protein metabolism. Important for healthy hair, skin, liver, and eyes.
Vitamin B_{12} ◊X	A wide variety of animal sources such as organ meats (beef liver), shellfish (clams), meat and poultry Fish like salmon, rainbow trout, light canned tuna Soybeans	Helps your body produce red blood cells and use fat and carbohydrates for energy.
B complex—Niacin	Peanuts Beef Chicken	Niacin is a type of B vitamin that helps the digestive system, skin, and nerves to function. Important for converting food to energy.
B complex—Riboflavin	Green leafy vegetables Eggs Legumes Lean meats Dairy products Nuts Mushrooms Zucchini Fortified cereals Beef liver	A type of B vitamin involved in energy metabolism.

X Important for pregnancy   ◊ Often found to be deficient in the elderly

NUTRIENT	FOOD SOURCE	NOTES
B complex—Thiamin	Pine nuts Soybeans Broccoli rabe	A type of B vitamin that helps turn carbohydrates into energy.
Vitamin C~	Oranges Red and green bell peppers Kale Broccoli Zucchini Cauliflower Brussels sprouts Papaya Strawberries Pineapple Mangoes Fennel Broccoli rabe Beets	An antioxidant and important for skin, bone, and connective tissue health. Promotes healing and helps the body absorb iron. Ascorbic acid (vitamin C) is added to cured meats to help prevent the carcinogen nitrosamine forming from nitrite.
Vitamin D*◊X~±	Sunshine Fish (especially fatty fishes like swordfish, salmon, and mackerel) Cod liver oil Soybeans Fortified foods and beverages like milk, OJ, cereal	Helps calcium absorption and bone growth.
Vitamin E◊~	Nuts Seeds Green leafy vegetables Broccoli rabe Wheat germ Fortified cereals	Powerful antioxidant Excessive levels can be dangerous for the elderly because of its anticoagulant property.

~ Important for babies   * Often found to be deficient in children
± Often found to be deficient in teens   ◊ Often found to be deficient in the elderly
X Important for pregnancy

NUTRIENT	FOOD SOURCE	NOTES
Vitamin K$^\lozenge$	Radicchio Green leafy vegetables like kale, spinach, collard greens Broccoli rabe Turnips Mustard greens Zucchini Leeks	Important for blood clotting
Zinc$^{*\sim}$	Whole grains (especially the germ and bran) Legumes Nuts Liver Meat Eggs Oysters Poultry Alaskan king crab	Shown to play a role in immune function.

~ Important for babies   * Often found to be deficient in children
$\lozenge$ Often found to be deficient in the elderly

UNIVERSAL CONVERSION CHART

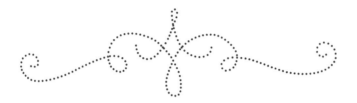

250°F = 120°C   350°F = 180°C   450°F = 230°C

275°F = 135°C   375°F = 190°C   475°F = 240°C

300°F = 150°C   400°F = 200°C   500°F = 260°C

325°F = 160°C   425°F = 220°C

MEASUREMENT EQUIVALENTS

Measurements should always be level unless directed otherwise.

⅛ teaspoon = 0.5 ml

¼ teaspoon = 1 ml

½ teaspoon = 2 ml

1 teaspoon = 5 ml

1 tablespoon = 3 teaspoons = ½ fluid ounce = 15 ml

2 tablespoons = ⅛ cup = 1 fluid ounce = 30 ml

4 tablespoons = ¼ cup = 2 fluid ounces = 60 ml

5⅓ tablespoons = ⅓ cup = 3 fluid ounces = 80 ml

8 tablespoons = ½ cup = 4 fluid ounces = 120 ml

10⅔ tablespoons = ⅔ cup = 5 fluid ounces = 160 ml

12 tablespoons = ¾ cup = 6 fluid ounces = 180 ml

16 tablespoons = 1 cup = 8 fluid ounces = 240 ml

INDEX

Note: Page references in *italics* refer to photos of recipes and ingredients.